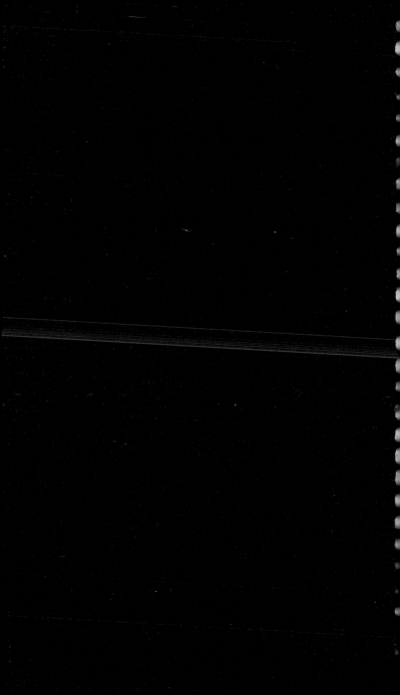

nh

'Lees takes the reader on an extraordinary journey inside and outside the brain. His deep humanity and honesty shines throughout. The inevitable comparison with the late, great Oliver Sacks is entirely just.' – Raymond Tallis

'Andrew Lees enters a powerful protest against the narrow, bureaucratic and often commercially-tainted nature of what is nowadays counted as evidence. He tells a fascinating story . . . and he pleads for much greater freedom for researchers to make leaps of the imagination in place of endless form-filling. If only the government would listen!' – Theodore Dalrymple, prison doctor and author of *Junk Medicine: Doctors, Lies and the Addiction Bureaucracy.*

'As medical research and practice gets squeezed by the iron hand of evidence based conformity, Andrew Lees celebrates the honourable tradition of the hunch in medical diagnosis and treatment.' – Professor John Hardy, winner of the 2015 Discovery Prize

'A fascinating and engrossing memoir that pays homage to the creative genius of the Beat Generation's most challenging writer, William S. Burroughs. This book redefines the relationship between doctors, drugs, and patients. A pleasure to read.' – Bill Morgan, Author of *I Celebrate Myself: The Somewhat Private Life of Allen Ginsber*g

Andrew Lees is a Professor of Neurology at the National Hospital, Queen Square London. He is the recipient of numerous awards including the American Academy of Neurology Life Time Achievement Award, the Association of British Neurologists' Medal, the Dingebauer Prize for Outstanding Research and the Gowers Medal. He is one of the three most highly cited Parkinson's disease researchers in the world. He is the author of several books, including *Ray of Hope*, runner-up in the William Hill Sports Book of the Year, *Hurricane Port* and *The Silent Plague*.

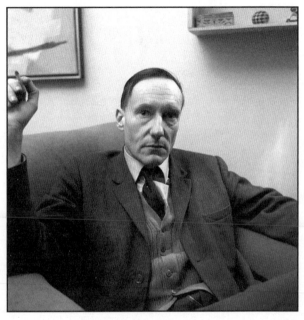

William Burroughs, London, 1960

A. J. Lees

–

MENTORED
BY A MADMAN

–

The William Burroughs Experiment

Notting Hill Editions

First published in 2016
by Notting Hill Editions Ltd
Widworthy Barton, Honiton, Devon EX14 9JS
This edition published in 2017.

Designed by FLOK Design, Berlin, Germany
Typeset by CB editions, London

Printed and bound
by Memminger MedienCentrum, Memmingen, Germany

A CIP record for this book
is available from the British Library

ISBN 978-1-910749-10-4

www.nottinghilleditions.com

Altamirage is that special personal quality by which good luck is prompted as a result of personally distinctive actions. In contrast, serendipity involves finding valuable things as a result of happy accidents, general exploratory behaviour, or sagacity. The most novel scientific discoveries occur when several varieties of chance coincide.

Contents

James Grauerholz

– Foreword –

'Doctorhood is being made with me'
– Dr Konstantins Raudive, *Breakthrough:
An Amazing Experiment in Electronic Communication
with the Dead* (1971)

The book in your hands was entirely written in the three years since I first met Dr Andrew Lees via email and we became pen pals. It is a compelling, unpredictable and quirky life-review, which everyone should read. And I would still make that statement even if this book were not as riddled as a raisin cake with the words and ideas of William S. Burroughs . . . which it certainly is! Thus, it is my sincere pleasure to commend it humbly to your attention.

Andrew and I first made contact when he asked his good friend, the late Dr Oliver Sacks, to put out word to Sacks' network that Lees was researching an article-in-progress, 'Hanging Out with the Molecules'. (That brief article, published in 2014 in the *Dublin Review of Books,* was in many ways Dr Lees' outline for this present work). At least two recipients of Sacks' emailing were old friends of mine and the late William S. Burroughs, whose companion I was and whose literary executor I am, so Andrew and I were soon in touch.

Captivated by Andrew's keen interest in all things Burroughs, I threw out lead after biographical lead, paths of research down the long years and documents of William's life – St Louis; Vienna; New York; Chicago; Paris – not counting the worlds of Burroughs' imagination, Interzones, that he rendered into his dozens of books and writings. (There are also many 'Doctor' figures to be seen among the prolific visual artworks that Burroughs made in his last decade).

Sometimes I can imagine Lees as the consummate Watson to Burroughs' Holmes; and, I rather think, so can Andrew – I know he is well-versed in the ways of Baker Street. Of course, Dr Watson always gave Sherlock Holmes all the credit for their successful cases, and my only reservation about *Mentored by a Madman* is that Andrew attributes so very much of his own medical insight to the effects on him of Burroughs' ideas.

Of course, even the most casual reader of Burroughs will know that, in his books, central roles are often played by medical and psychiatric doctors, neurosurgeons and nurses. Doctor Benway of *Naked Lunch,* in particular, has reached iconic status by now; but doctors and psychiatrists are *everywhere* in Burroughs' writings . . . like the familiar host of tiny, surreal, demon-figures who always gambol in the margins of the eschatological landscapes of Hieronymus Bosch.

The key to this 'mentorship' is that Lees and Burroughs never met in person: it was etheric, and intergenerational. Already, in Lees' career as a young doctor, the Burroughsian Word Virus was helping to light the way toward his own discoveries and innovations.

So was Burroughs really a madman? It has always been easy enough to see the mature author and his auto-protagonist that way, from a distance. Many of his literary doctors are 'mad doctors', a character type that he did not originate but to which he memorably added. His biography and his mythos did not dispel his own mad-doctor impression.

William's friends will agree that it is undoubtedly very much for the best that he dropped out of his medical classes at the Universitaet Wien. Burroughs loved to *imagine* himself a doctor, but surely, many future patients' lives were spared by that lucky turn of events in Austria in the winter of 1936–7.

And yet those horrific months in the notorious Dr Eduard Pernkopf's anatomy class, and young Burroughs' other medical studies, have given us such immortal characters as:

Dr Tetrazzini – who does not so much operate as *perform*:

I say perform advisedly because his operations were performances. He would start by throwing a scalpel across the room into the patient and then make his entrance like a ballet dancer. His speed was incredible: 'I don't give them time to die,' he would say. Tumors put him in a frenzy of rage. 'Fucking undisciplined cells!' he would snarl, advancing on the tumor like a knife-fighter.'

Doctor Benway, who says to his students,

'Now, boys, you won't see this operation performed very often and there's a reason for that . . . You see it has absolutely no medical value . . . I think it was a pure artistic creation from the beginning.'

And the German Practitioner of Technical Medicine:

'The human body is filled up vit unnecessary parts. They should not be so close in together crowded. You can get by vit von kidney. Vy have two?' [And he adds, *sotto voce,* peering ominously into the abdominal cavity:] 'Yes dot is a kidney . . .'

And then with a straight face, there is William himself, solemnly pontificating to me that, since he never got a cold when he had a junk habit, therefore the junk must be delivering a protective antiviral coating to his cells. I told him: 'Maybe it's because on junk you never leave your house, so how could you even catch a virus.' Oh, we had fun.

The heart of this book is that Andrew Lees has, all his career, taken on board the peculiar potpourri of visionary ideas and crackpot theories that come from 'the mad Burroughs'. Unlike most of his contemporaries in neurology, Dr Lees gave Burroughs the benefit of the doubt, and asked himself the scientist's indispensable questions: Why not? And what if?

Science – 'pure science' – relies for the solidity of

its intellectual edifice on proofs, excluded middles, logical certainty and the like. But without experiment, there is no theory . . . and when Burroughs in 1953 was in a *brujo's* shack in the rotting jungle under a full moon, drinking a cup of black, oily, fresh-brewed yage-vine liquor with no assurance of his safety or even survival, that was *experimental.*

The truth is out there. You want to believe. And if you are so lucky, perhaps you broaden the healing arts. I speak of the art of science, of art *as* science – not of misguided 'scientism', nor all the Faustian terrors of our modern age. These 20th-century dysfunctions were diagnosed early by the West's bohemian post-War generation, weren't they . . . for what *is* Beat Mind in the first place, but forms of that same 'madness' by which Allen Ginsberg in *Howl*, 1956, saw 'the great minds of [his] generation . . . destroyed'? And then the sacralization of that madness, all madness, recuperated from the doctor-authorities and claimed by the mad, for the mad, *détourné*, Occupied, contested.

As Andrew Lees' life story shows, he enjoys an endearing immunity to whatever it is that makes doctors overbearing and under-bearable. He does see himself seriously as a committed healer, upholding his oaths Hippocratic and Aesculapeian . . .

'Of course, he has his *ethical standards* . . .' – as William might sardonically quip.

But hold the irony, because I do believe it has been neurology's good fortune that Andrew Lees can also see some of himself in old Doctor Benway, making that first appearance in Cambridge, Massachusetts, 1938, with William and his best friend from St Louis, Kells Elvins, co-writing 'Twilight's Last Gleamings':

'S. S. America, off Jersey coast' . . . Explosion splits the boat . . .

By the dawn's early light, Dr. Benway, Ship's Doctor, pushed through a crowd at the rail and boarded the first life-boat.

'Are you all alright?' he said, seating himself among the women . . .

'I'm the Doctor.'

Kansas, 5 February 2016

– Preface –

In a medical field where there are so many brutal and incurable diseases, research designed to find remedies should be an integral part of the duty of care. Thirty years ago this was accepted and encouraged in neurology. Barriers have now been erected between the universities and the National Health Service that have created serious deterrents to clinical research. Academics, who sometimes prefer to call themselves clinical neuroscientists rather than neurologists, spend more and more time in their offices writing large grant applications, calculating their own impact based on their publications, and dreaming of the chimera of bench to bedside.

Neurologists have a calling and live a great part of their lives in the cloisters of the hospital. Like the police, we prefer our own company. The centenary of William Burroughs' birth in 2014 was the spur I needed to let the cat out of the bag. It was not censure by the authorities or damage to my reputation that delayed the writing of this book but a fear of ostracism by my colleagues. To be cast out by the brotherhood would have been a punishment far greater than imprisonment.

I had realised during casual conversations over the years that few neurologists had even heard of William Burroughs let alone read him. *Naked Lunch*, his best-known work, was not on the recommended reading list for aspiring medical students. The few who had read Burroughs told me that they found most of it unintelligible and his diatribes against doctors and scientists deluded.

William Burroughs would have made a dreadful neurologist but he helped me to find some of the answers my patients craved, and sustained my curiosity for self-experimentation. He understood the secret of fascination. He was a virus in the dogma, the extraterrestrial in the ointment, the third that walked beside me and influenced some of my most lasting achievements. He taught me a method of inquiry that depended on divine secret and unnoticed features. Eventually I came to see his crazy pronouncements as a Hippocratic Oath for Medical Science.

Too much is omitted and forgotten and too much imagined for this to be a memoir. I prefer to call it a fantasia. The story is a far cry from the glorious blood and thunderous craft of brain surgery and the hardcore molecular science of the wet laboratory. It is an idiosyncratic botany trip along the backwaters of observational research. It is a plea for open-mindedness and freedom.

The Hargreaves Building, Liverpool, 2016

– Synchronicity –

On October 5 1982, whilst I was preparing for an interview for the most senior position of my career, William Seward Burroughs entered a Liverpool that was still tense after the Toxteth riots. A small promotion tucked away in the *Echo* was the only public announcement:

A MAN OF INFLUENCE

Waiting for the man? William Burroughs, divine mentor, legend etc., whose books have influenced people like Lou Reed, Patti Smith, David Bowie and many others comes to Liverpool tonight for a rare reading of his works. Time 7-30pm. Be there early or the cult following will get all the seats.

Geoff Ward, a young university lecturer in English Literature, was there to welcome his hero at Lime Street Station with a gift of a bottle of vodka. Burroughs was polite but there was no small talk. Ensconced in the Adelphi Hotel, Burroughs idly turned the television on and sat immersed in a documentary on lemurs. His penumbral presence sucked the oxygen from the room and created an echo chamber. He had fallen out of the world into himself and was almost invisible, dematerialised but for the cold-blooded glow of his eyes. As the afternoon dragged on, an aromatic whiff of weed floated down the long, empty second-floor corridor. His large entourage including one man making kerpow noises with an imitation gun, ignored the insistent knocking on the door by a chambermaid dressed in full burlesque attire.

That evening Burroughs did a signing at the Atticus bookshop on Hardman Street. He was courteous and eager to socialise. A scally handed him a Tarzan comic, which he autographed without blinking an eye. He complimented the management on a terrific display that included issue 4/5 of *Re/Search* magazine in which he featured on the front cover. Inside was an article in which he talked about his advanced ideas about the social control process. He then walked over to the Conference Hotel accompanied by James Grauerholz, John Giorno of Dial-a-Poem fame, ex-Warhol disciple Victor Bockris and Roger Ely, one of the organisers with Genesis P-Orridge of the Final Academy, a series of events featuring Burroughs that had taken place at the Ritzy Cinema in Brixton and the Hacienda Club in Manchester.

The deliberately chosen cheap and neutral venue situated on Mount Pleasant had recently hosted the Liverpool finals of the Miss Caribbean contest. About a hundred and fifty arty punks sat in silent anticipation. Ward, who had described the events of the day to me, plucked up courage to ask Burroughs what he felt about dying, to which the tortured response had come: 'Well it's a step in the right direction'.

The 'happening' began with poetry readings by Adrian Henri of the Liverpool Scene, Geoff Ward and Jeff Nuttall, one of the first Englishmen to champion Burroughs in *My Own Mag* in the sixties. These understated, low-key British performances were followed by a full-on bellowing rendition of 'Just Say No to Family Values' by the American performance poet John Giorno.

Then Burroughs got up. 'Can you all hear me?' he drawled in his funereal voice. He began by reading extracts from his new book, *The Place of Dead Roads*. He explained that a 'Johnson' was a harmless person who kept his word and honoured his obligations, minded his own business and would not stand by to watch innocent people die. He was the polar opposite of a 'Shit' – a sanctimonious hypocrite who craved power and tried to enforce his harmful viewpoint on others. Shits comprised about one fifth of the American population and were responsible for all that was wrong in the world. He next introduced his protagonist, the gunslinging gay junky Kim Carsons whose mission was to organise the Johnson family into a worldwide space programme. Carsons was a morbid, slimy youth of unwholesome proclivities with an insatiable appetite for the extreme and the sensational who adored ectoplasm and crystal balls. He stank like a polecat and wallowed in abomination.

Burroughs next launched into a folkloric text related to his experiences in the Lexington Narcotics Hospital. The 'do rights' were sycophantic inmates who had acquired good bedside manners and who pretended they had made their peace with Jesus and the star-spangled banner in a cynical attempt to squeeze more dope from their gullible doctors.

He concluded the reading with an extract from 'Twilights Last Gleamings', a story he had written together with his childhood friend Kells Elvins, in which the first mention of Doctor Benway appears:

Dr. Benway, ships doctor, drunkenly added two inches to a four-inch incision with one stroke of his scalpel.

'Perhaps the appendix is already out doctor?' The nurse said. Appearing dubiously over his shoulder, 'I saw a little scar.'

'The appendix already out!'

'I'm taking the appendix out!'

'What do you think I'm doing here?!'

'Perhaps the appendix is on the left side doctor that happens sometimes you know!'

'Stop breathing down my neck I'm coming to that.'

'Don't you think I know where an appendix is?'

'I studied appendectomy in 1904 at Harvard.'

Burroughs' performance was animated, polished and wickedly humorous despite the fact he had been smoking dope all day and drinking red wine and vodka since late afternoon. He had travelled sideways into myth and backwards into history to reveal contemporary phantoms. He released an atom-deep sensation of otherworldliness on a Liverpool scene.

On the same day Burroughs arrived in Liverpool for the first and only time, I was successfully appointed to the post of Consultant Neurologist to the National Hospital for Nervous Diseases, Queen Square and University College Hospital in London. I had toed the line, avoided making powerful enemies and had endeavoured to develop a dignified uniformity with my fellow man. Despite my retiring and solitary nature, a flair for clinical research had carried me home. I also had a wife and two small children that helped to falsely reassure the interview panel that I was unlikely to be a deviant or subversive. I was relieved not to have lost out to opponents that I considered less deserving, yet the burden of responsibility that came with this new office filled me with fear. I had now joined the Establishment and would find it much harder to challenge authority.

William Burroughs had been my dark angel and cultural guru since our intersection at medical school and Liverpool was the eternal city of my childhood that I could never leave behind. The events of October 5, 1982, were a concatenation and became an expression of a deeper intuitive order.

As I had gone through my training I had learned to treat the person not the disease. William Osler's words 'Ask not what disease the person has but rather what person the disease has' had become my modus operandi. I had come to understand the importance of the nuanced explanation, the calm gesture and the reassuring smile. I had observed my patients' varied responses to their treatment and grasped the mystery of the therapeutic process.

I tried as best I could to enter into my patients' mode of thought. I avoided at all costs saying to them, 'I understand how you feel'. Many of my decisions were now based on informed guesses, hunches and imaginings; exploratory acts motivated by a passion to do good and quite independent of scientific knowledge. Unconscious wisdom, know-how and rules of thumb all played a part in my doctoring. I looked at the wider picture and when I felt it appropriate I self-experimented to obtain answers. I did my best to relieve suffering and preserve health but most of all I wanted to find new cures.

From now on, William Burroughs would be my guiding lamp. He was Dr Henry Jekyll warning me about hubris, the power of imagery and the dangers of regulation. I needed to verify, refute and establish the validity of everything I did in relation to the sour smell of nervous disease. Every effect had its cause and there was no such thing as a coincidence. There was no turning back. I was hooked on unreality.

2

– Doctor Benway –

An encyclopaedic knowledge of redundant ports and a passion for grasses and trees contrived to launch me on a career in medicine. My schoolboy geography did not revolve around mountain ranges or capitals but focused on entrepôts like Manaus where rare flowers waited in boxes to be dispatched to Liverpool. I liked to focus on those spaces on maps marked *terra incognita* and small mysterious islands like Terceira in the Azores. My history reading glossed over battles, treaties, and the lives of England's monarchs but focused on the lives of the great naval explorers like Álvaro Cabral and Amerigo Vespucci. These adventurers who had made journeys into the unknown became my honorary ancestors.

A year after I had passed my GCE O-level examinations I was asked to attend for interview at the London Hospital Medical College in Whitechapel. The train journey from Leeds took me past arable land alive with fluttering peewits, cooling towers and northern ings littered with the feathers of mutilated swans. At the Kings Cross depôt I entered the zigzag of underground corridors and stairs that led me to the Tube.

I was now in an after world of perpetual solitude,

another level down, above the tombs with nothing to worry about. The Underground train doors closed shut and we careered through endless echoing darkness, drawing in air before finally breaking cover in the Whitechapel cutting. I felt like a diminutive package in a canister being sucked through an airless system of pipes.

I alighted on Platform 4, climbed the wide flight of stairs and walked across the overhead bridge that linked the station's islands to the booking office. Rows of market stalls with the bluster of Jewish costermongers greeted me on the Whitechapel Road. 'Blame it on the Bossa Nova' (the dance of love) by Eydie Gormé, was blasting out from Paul's for Music. Across the road emblazoned on a large yellow brick building below a huge clock with its round stone bezel and ashen face were the words 'The London Hospital'. In the anaemic sunlight I stared up at the attic where Joseph Merrick, 'The Elephant Man', had first found peace.

I climbed the stairs to the hospital, walked through its imposing colonnade and past the forecourt full of parked Daimlers and ambulances. At the lodge in the front wing, the dapper head porter pointed me in the direction of a short flight of stairs that led to the Board Room. A middle-aged woman dressed in a prim blouse told me to take a seat outside the door. I rehearsed again the extracts I had memorised from the College prospectus. The London Infirmary, later to become The London Hospital, had been founded by six businessmen in the Feathers Tavern in 1740, primarily for the relief of all sick merchant seamen. It had later become the first voluntary hospital to offer a teaching course of lectures as well as an apprenticeship. According to my mother, who had thoroughly researched the hospital's credentials, diseases of the poor and exotic maladies common in lascars were its particular forte.

After a short delay I was ushered in by the secretary and asked to sit on a hard backed chair without arms. I explained to my ten genial inquisitors that for the last three years I had kept diaries of garden birds and had learned the importance of accurate observation and precise recording through contact with learned men in the Leeds Naturalist's Club. As the interview was drawing to an end, I raised one or two chuckles from the committee when I told them that 'The London' was my first choice because of its proximity to the docks. The chairman, Dr John Ellis, then stood up and thanked me for attending. As I left the room I could see two of the committee members smiling conspiratorially.

In less than a minute I was back out on the Whitechapel Road under a clay white sky. I slipped down the stairs of the Underground as if it was a ship's ladder. On the way back to Kings Cross, I started to enjoy the contingencies between the train stopping and the doors opening. The noise of a passing car on the other line recalled Atlantic breakers. The slamming of the doors sounded like a giant wave of surf rolling down the platform. I was in deep and a long way from shore.

Two weeks later my parents received a short note informing them I had been offered a place on the proviso that I didn't flunk my A-levels. None of the doctors and surgeons on the panel had asked me if there were doctors in the family, whether I played rugby for the school first team, or if I could recall whether stethoscopes and nurses had featured in my childhood play routines. My destiny had been sealed in less than half an hour but for now I could keep my distance and return to the neutrality and beauty of nature. I kept returning to the Liverpool Landing Stage to look out at that exotic grey horizon. The Manaus riverboats haunted my dreams.

I arrived back in Whitechapel eighteen months later on October 4, 1965 to begin my apprenticeship. My year was composed of a mix of public school and grammar school entrants from all over the United Kingdom but only seven out of the eighty were women and there were no black students. In his welcome address, the Dean informed us that we were here to study medicine and that from now on our lives would be dedicated to the prevention, cure or alleviation of human disease. Medicine was a calling, not a business. He hoped that we would all live up to the high traditions of our chosen profession and represent 'The London' with honour and trustworthiness. *Homo sum, humani nihil a me alienum puto* – 'I am a human being, I consider nothing that is human foreign to me' was the hospital's motto.

On my third day, I lined up in embarrassment with Lampard, Lashman, Lawford, Lewin and Lupini by the side of the last dead body on the row of cadavers. A smell of rancid sickliness tinged with the pungency of fixative turned our stomachs. Our corpse was a man called Wolynski, portly, with a gargantuan head and sparse body hair. His name tag stated that he had died of natural causes nine months earlier. I imagined he must have been a Polish seaman who had collapsed in a boarding house down by the river. He was a stunning figurine waiting to be vandalised. My first cut into his swollen arm revealed a morass of deathly beigeness devoid of the glistening red, white and blue of living flesh. Soon Wolynski became little more than a giant rat.

I had been forced to accept that a career collecting rare flowers in an imaginary homeland was now no more than an adolescent dream and my focus transferred to the anatomy of the human body. I applied ribald mnemonics to the tributaries of the carotid artery and reduced the brachial plexus to roots, trunks and branches. Our surgical demonstrator Andrew Paris took us to the museum where we pored over pots of pickled organs under the watchful eye of Merrick's skeleton. Paris told us we were embarking on an adventure that may take us to places beyond our mind's eye.

I shut myself away in my room to memorise Henry

Gray's descriptions and recite the name of each ridge and groove of my second-hand bone collection. I wrote home to reassure my anxious parents that I was adjusting to leaving home and enjoying medical school. Fortunately, my mother had not got wind of the fact that a doctor's son from Wales had shot himself in the first week of term, reducing our number to seventy-nine. But my letters did not really tell the truth. London was a different country and a faceless monster that both excited and frightened me. I desperately missed those kindly flat vowels and people who talked to me at bus stops. I missed the passion and romance of little Northern towns like St Helens, Widnes, Wigan and Oldham and the intergalactic highway of Liverpool. I had closed down and curled inwards. Study had become a pathetic solace and a remedy for homesickness.

When our picking was finally complete, Wolynski's frozen remains were removed from the dissection room and buried. His 'cutting open' had been our rite of passage. A rumour that passed from one generation of students to the next was that at the end of each term the mauled cadavers were transported on a dead body train from the hospital to Whitechapel Station and then to a place of rest near the necropolis of Brick Lane. I was not invited to Wolynski's funeral but I was grateful for his sacrifice and have never forgotten him. He had helped me to acquire the carapace of insensitivity required to become a doctor.

Once I had negotiated the 2nd MB examinations in physiology, anatomy, human biochemistry and clinical pharmacology and become a clinical dresser on Sister Paulin's Ward, I relaxed my studying a little. I found conversing with the sick distressing and nerve-racking. I lacked confidence and felt inept, particularly when I had to present cases on teaching rounds. Some of the patients' stories were harrowing and I marvelled at their bravery in the face of serious illness. The gentleness and solicitude of many of the student nurses embarrassed me. In their mauve and white checked dresses with puffed sleeves, separate white buttoned collars and starched aprons they glided like seraphim between the bays. Changing colostomy bags and lifting dead weights took love and selflessness.

It was around this time that I started Harlem shuffling with a cool yé-yé crowd at Le Kilt, Birdland and Le Bataclan in Soho. I was all dressed up with a pair of grey striped hipster flares, Ravel shoes and a skin-tight ribbed crew neck sweater worn over a blue crepe shirt. The chic French au pairs wore very short kilts, tight Shetlands and plenty of black pencil. I was out on a limb, an 'in crowd' modernist leading a double life. I was navigating between alternate worlds.

Some Sunday afternoons I would walk from Stepney Way across Commercial Road through a wasteland of bloodshed and beer down to Limehouse and Poplar past the now deserted West India Docks. I was drawn towards the river, the dock road and the Isle of Dogs.

I wished to be at home and away simultaneously. It seemed as if I was always in another place, dancing and mourning.

After these break-outs I returned to my textbooks with renewed commitment. If study had gone well that week, I would go out again in the evening for a half pint in The Grave Maurice. On the other side of its beguiling velvet curtain there were diamond geezers with flashy broads bathed in subdued light. I loved the affectionate way the Cockneys talked to me, their rhyming slang, their unaffected cosmopolitanism, and above all, their sense of community. In these casual encounters I was acutely aware of my provinciality and slow-wittedness.

By Monday morning the two halves of London that never added up to a whole were forgotten, as I assisted in theatre, delivered babies at Mile End and navigated the long frightening corridors of the Claybury asylum. My neurology and psychiatry teachers galvanised me and in spare moments I went to the College library to read up on motor neurone disease and brain tumours. In Enoch and Trethowan's *Uncommon Psychiatric Syndromes* I learned that Cotard's was a delusional disorder in which the sufferer believed he was a walking corpse and that De Clérembault's was a disabling, obsessive, unrequited love.

The teaching autopsy too was an eagerly anticipated ritual. Our medical firm (Bomford and Ellis) would troop across the road from the hospital to the mortuary where a clinician would present the history and physical signs of the deceased and then the morbid anatomists, under the watchful eye of Professor 'Doe' (Doniach) would reveal the macroscopic pathological findings. Henry Urich, perched on a ledge next to the cadaver, would lead the discussion on the neurological cases in his intense Eastern European accent as we hung spellbound on his every word. Urich used a large knife to skilfully cut open the brain on what looked like a large breadboard. The naked-eye appearance of the coronally sliced hemispheres and the transverse cuts of the brain stem allowed him to suspect diagnoses such as Parkinson's disease. With the help of a large pair of toothless forceps he magically exposed other pathologies, such as water on the brain, neoplasms, obscure degenerations and catastrophic haemorrhage. These demonstrations taught me the great level of uncertainty relating to the cause of death in so many autopsies, the common occurrence of more than one pathology in the elderly and most importantly of all, the need for humility in medicine. Urich also reminded us that there were more secrets waiting to be revealed when the fixed brain was examined under the light microscope.

This new knowledge I was acquiring as a medical student re-ignited my interest in the world of living creatures but also inspired a new fascination with dead matter. Human life in its development and decay, with its ever-varied patterns of disease, presented me with new dilemmas of the highest interest. There seemed to be a great deal of advantage of coming in at the end of the story when all the facts were in. Pathology gave me security.

But just when I started to feel I was getting to grips with my training, a disturbing sense of disaffection reared up. Most of my peers now seemed self-satisfied and narrow-minded. Carrying out a vaginal examination in theatre on an anaesthetised woman with fibroids without her prior consent, seemed even then like an assault. Being told by the registrar to go and see 'the gastric cancer in the big end' seemed crude and inhumane. On electives to other hospitals, such as my short time at the overcrowded South Ockenden Institute for Mental Defectives, I felt that care was too often casual and matter-of-fact and that most of the severely handicapped patients had been stripped of their dignity. I didn't blame the nurses as much as a system that lacked a will for change. Then I was ordered by Sister Gloucester to get my shoulder-length hair cut before she would let me back on her ward. My reluctance to comply was a feeble and selfish expression of growing rebellion. I became increasingly sensitive to judgmental condescension. Received Pronunciation was expected and my Northern English accent was scorned and imitated by some of my peers and teachers.

It was the front cover of the Beatles' *Sergeant Pepper's Lonely Hearts Club Band* that first brought William Burroughs into view. Amidst the rows of famous faces he was on the second row next to Marilyn Monroe and above Oscar Wilde. I didn't recognise him so I looked him up.

I learned that Burroughs was in his own words a 'queer', who after 'accidentally' shooting his common law wife, Joan Vollmer, in Mexico City had fled to Colombia in search of a telepathic truth drug called yagé. His lurid descriptions of heroin-laced depravity, sodomy and infanticide in *Naked Lunch* had been described by a Boston judge as 'a revolting miasma of unrelieved perversion'. A connection with Paul McCartney and Barry Miles at the Indica bookshop had got him on the cover. He seemed to have come out of nowhere.

The conformity of medicine was suffocating me. There seemed more interesting things to do than playing bridge in the Students Union, going to 'hops' on Wednesday evenings or singing Zulu warrior after a rugby game at Hale End. The medical establishment was still dominated by old school ties and funny handshakes. Subjects that seemed important to me, like the management of drug addiction or the rudiments of forensic medicine, did not appear anywhere on the medical student curriculum. I began to harbour reservations whether unconditionally helping the sick was going to be sufficiently fulfilling for the next fifty years.

One day in November 1969, in rebellious mood I got hold of a Corgi paperback copy of *Naked Lunch*.

The front cover had a stark image of Burroughs with eerie red irises and a blotchy cut-up montage that included a face and a monkey superimposed on his forehead. It suggested pulp detective fiction but the first lines had a spooky authority:

I can feel the heat closing in, feel them out there making their moves, setting up their devil doll stool pigeons, crooning over my spoon and dropper I throw away at Washington Square Station, vault a turnstile and two flights down the iron stairs, catch an uptown A train . . .

Naked Lunch was hard-boiled, clinical and detached, its characters shadowy and glacial with hollow voices. Burroughs told his readers that you could cut into its text at any intersection point; there was no beginning or end, just an infinite stream of consciousness. Reality and dream were illusory and neither could exist without the other. It was a mosaic of depravity, violence and cruelty driven by plain sexual desire, the Grim Reaper's very own missive from Hell.

It was also a tour through the school urinals with the musty smell of stale wank and jock straps and a prelude to my urology surgical dressership with descriptions of bifurcated penises, ejaculation on hanging (angel lust), and priapism. Burroughs' writing spilt off the page in all directions and wallowed in excrement. It was a far cry from the drama of the kitchen sink.

Doc Benway, the darkly comical Director of the

Freeland Reconditioning Centre, made me laugh. He was an amalgam of all the bastard doctors Burroughs had ever encountered: the blinkered New York shrinks, the reckless blundering St Louis surgeons and the Mexico City prescription-forgers. Benway had been recruited as an advisor to the Republic of Freeland, a country given over to free love and communal bathing, and reputedly based on Scandinavia. Homosexuality is considered an infectious disease and in his laboratory he carries out aversive experiments on heterosexual rats that turn them into 'fruit rats'.

Benway's unsettling bedside manner reminded me of my surgical teacher CT's old-school gentlemanly demeanour combined with his penchant for drastic and fearless intervention. His punitive ward rounds, where terrified juniors and a simpering nursing sister would lead him on a sight-seeing tour of his condemned lung cancer victims, were an abomination. Many of his operated patients were in severe pain but nevertheless were expected to sit bolt upright in bed as the great man strode by. He rarely spoke directly to his patients. In theatre he threw scalpels and humiliated his assistants. His power was absolute and his decision-making infallible. He gave the impression that he had a visceral contempt for the frailty of the human organism.

CT was a frightening hero renowned for his icy silences. There were several other practitioners and craftsmen with similar reputations at The London Hospital. A houseman on another of the general surgery wards told me how he had been forced to devise strategies to keep his boss away from incurable and dying patients' colons. On ward rounds I learned the expression frequently used by surgeons that 'the operation had been a technical success but the patient had died', implying it was the anaesthetist who had committed manslaughter.

Doc. Benway was medicine's arch-enemy, a villain without a first name addicted to mind control surgery. He was enamoured by the abstract scientific process and unconcerned about who owned his research findings – he was on a quest for knowledge for its own sake. At Claybury Hospital, on my psychiatry elective, I saw insulin coma therapy, electro convulsive treatment and prefrontal leucotomies used to subdue the mentally ill but Benway's fascination with electrical brain stimulators was still in the realms of science fiction. His mastery of brainwashing techniques, widely employed by the KGB and CIA, was all that was needed for now. This subversion of the medical model appealed to my rebellious streak. Benway was an operative of the State employed to find new ways of creating automatic obedience.

Some of the black humour in *Naked Lunch* was implanted in my impressionable brain, along with textbook descriptions of diseases I had never seen:

'They have no feelings,' said Doctor Benway, slashing his patient to shreds.

Did I ever tell you about the time I performed an appendectomy with a rusty sardine can? And once I was caught short without instrument one and removed a uterine tumor with my teeth.

Benway's confabs with his colleague Dr Schafer, the Lobotomy Kid, about creating a talking asshole that would improve human efficiency, were a chilling preview of a brave new world of genetic engineering, and his electrical stimulation of the mind did eventually become a surgical reality. Benway was grey and faceless and strode between Hippocrates and I, a disturbing third presence who could help me fail finals and free up time.

London now dragged like an anchor. Burroughs had convinced me that rationality could only ever rule part of our minds. The phantasmagorical description of the Composite City in *Naked Lunch*, filled with infernal scenes and foreign landscapes, was the London where I now lived. Burroughs had opened a crystal door that led to the moon.

3

– Magic Bullet –

My first house physician's appointment was at St Stephen's Hospital (now the Chelsea and Westminster Hospital) on the Fulham Road, where an acute 'medical take' consisted of five or six self-poisonings with sleeping pills like Mogadon and Mandrax, and a couple of bad LSD trips. Most of the 'attempted suicides' lived in bedsits and seemed to be seeking a holiday from the tedium of their mundane existence. A few had got into a mess and needed referral to the new breed of medical social workers that had displaced the hospital almoner. I was trying to get some proper medical experience under my belt and found it hard to be sympathetic. All I was doing was mopping up the wreckage of Swinging London.

Blomfield, the Casualty Officer, had hair down to his back, called me 'man' over the phone and wore *Release* and *CND* badges on the lapel of his white coat. The disorientated dialogue of some of the addicts we talked down late at night reminded me of the string of disjointed 'sets' in *Naked Lunch*.

In striking contrast to my 'take nights' in the newly built Accident and Emergency Department, the long wards in the old hospital were full of very ill elderly people with pneumonia, cancer and dropsy, collectively referred to in the doctor's mess as 'crumble'. I spent most of my mornings listening to their tales and ordering blood tests, electrocardiograms and chest X rays. Many were comfortably off but unlike the closely-knit East Enders they were isolated and lonely. When the time came for their hospital discharge, some didn't want to leave. I prescribed heroin to palliate severe pain in the dying and Guinness as a bedtime tonic, but kindness and cheerfulness were my most effective nostrums.

I had been in post for just three months when an elderly man who had worked on the London Underground was admitted from home. Parkinson's disease had confined him to a wheelchair and he was now dependent on his family to feed, dress and bathe him. The first telltale symptoms had started six years earlier when he had noticed an occasional quiver of the middle finger of the right hand when collecting tickets at Fulham Broadway. Within a year, stiffness and awkwardness in his hands had forced him to retire. He could now only take a few shuffling steps and his handwriting had been reduced to an illegible spidery scribble. Saliva dribbled constantly from the right side of his mouth and both his hands quaked interminably.

His reptilian stare suggested coldness and fear but he spoke warmly of his grandchildren and about his great love of pigeon racing. When he tried to take a few steps, he mumbled that it was like walking through treacle. He had told his wife that Parkinson's was a death sentence and that he was pinning all his hopes on the 'Dope'. He had read in the paper that the symptoms of Parkinson's disease could now be countered by an amino acid called L-3-4-dihydroxyphenylalanine (L-DOPA) that worked by boosting the brain's depleted levels of dopamine.

Parkinson's disease is the commonest neurological cause of chronic physical handicap in the elderly. It affects at least one in a hundred individuals over the age of sixty-five but can also strike down much younger people. The cause of the malady is not known but one interesting finding is that it is twice as common in non-smokers as cigarette smokers. It usually begins with maladroitness in one hand, aches and pains in an arm and feelings of tiredness. Some of those affected are at first thought by their families to be depressed, fatigued or to have become old overnight. The emergence of a tremble is the sign that cannot be ignored and usually leads to specialist referral. A loss of sense of smell, uncharacteristic maudlin eruptions, constipation and the acting out of dreams (rapid eye movement (REM) sleep disorder) are recognised prodromes. If Parkinson's disease is left untreated it deteriorates relentlessly, causing a quiet slurred speech, a hurrying shuffling gait and frequent falls. Progressive frailty, immobility and delirium lead to death within ten years of the first signs of the disease.

Slowness and stiffness, which are the most

disabling symptoms, are caused by severe damage to a small cluster of nerve cells called the substantia nigra (black stuff) located at the top of the brain stem. Under the microscope some of the remaining pigmented neurones contain bull's eye inclusions called Lewy bodies which allow the pathologist to confirm the diagnosis after death.

L-DOPA is a molecule found naturally in the pods of broad beans and in the pulses of the cowhage plant, a climbing legume used for centuries in Ayurvedic medicine. After it has been swallowed, it is actively absorbed in the upper gut and then transported by the blood stream, where a large quantity is broken down and excreted in the urine. A small proportion eventually crosses the blood-brain barrier and is then converted to dopamine. This Trojan horse approach to neurotransmitter replenishment is necessary because dopamine itself is not able to enter the brain.

After routine investigations had been completed, I started my new patient on three large white tablets of neat L-DOPA (*Larodopa*) and over the next ten days gradually increased the dose up to 3 grams a day. The nurses were instructed to take his blood pressure lying flat and then standing up every four hours and report any changes in his mobility to me.

On the fourth day it was obvious that his face had begun to thaw and he had started to blink again. After a week of L-DOPA he could use a knife and fork on his own and his voice had become much bolder. His handwriting doubled in size and no longer sloped upwards. On the tenth day he got out of his chair unaided and shuffled to the end of the ward. By the time he left hospital he had regained much of his independence. Parkinson's disease had taken away movements that it had taken him a lifetime to learn. He told me that he felt as if he had cast off a heavy space suit and an iron mask and come back to life.

L-DOPA had by now been heralded as a miracle cure but there had also been some sensational adverse headlines in the newspapers like, 'New drug makes sick old man chase nurses round the ward'. There were concerns that this unprecedented sudden return of mobility to chronically paralysed patients could trigger falls and unmask angina pectoris. These negative reports gained the medicine an early, unwarranted reputation as being unsafe and difficult to use.

For many years after its discovery, dopamine had been considered an inert intermediary on the synthetic pathway of the 'fight and flight' chemical messengers noradrenaline and adrenaline, and of no biological importance. By the early 1960s it was beginning to be more widely accepted that it was a chemical messenger and that its deficiency in the substantia nigra and corpus striatum (the basal ganglia) was responsible for the slowness and stiffness of Parkinson's disease. It was also now understood that the tranquilisers that had been found to be helpful in managing schizophrenia blocked dopamine receptors and could cause parkinsonism and depression as unwanted side effects.

The miracle of L-DOPA had turned me into 'Molecule Man' overnight. I was certain that further peptide and amine research would lead to cures for Alzheimer's disease and all the other brutal brain de-generations within five years.

4

– Looking for Clues –

A human brain looks like any other. Once it has been removed from the calvarium and the lining peeled away, it is a squelchy blancmange that dimples and blushes to the touch. After it has been fixed heavy with formalin it is putty in the hand, but holding it still feels momentous. It is not difficult to imagine that the walnut kernel I now rest on my palms used to spend hours watching ships sail down the river and was gifted in remembering faces. It is subtly asymmetrical with an intricate array of shiny fractals. From the sky its convolutions resemble a marshy wetland at low tide. There is no need to destroy it in order to communicate with the still life buried inside.

Optical microscopy first drew me to the brain's true beauty. Under high power magnification its silvered nerve cells resemble black leafless trees that have put down arborescent roots in the grey matter. Through my eyepiece I see climbing vines, grassy tufts, mossy tendrils and spiny shrubs. I observe how the pathology of Alzheimer's disease spreads like a forest fire leaving behind it desolate tumbleweed glades and how Parkinson's disease deposits ghost sunflower heads and twiners in the bleached nigra. Each sliver of inert tissue that becomes my focus appears like a microcosm of the Amazon valley. Inflorescences of unimaginable beauty nourished by rivulets of blood fill the gaps left by the dead trees. Dopamine and serotonin are the fluorescent butterflies of the soul, the sentimental amines that can never quite be pinned down. I am exploring death in inner space far below the brain's surface.

What I discover now alters constantly. Some of the trunks are draped with glial lianas. Ferns, air plants with rosaceous endings and dendritic thorns give way to an unforgettable flower-strewn landscape and then to an indefinable wood in which every charcoal tree is interconnected. I watch the forest metamorphose into an orchard of twiggy nerves and dying hyacinths. Empty, inaudible, and finally undone, the brain dissolves in the dim light and as I continue to pore down the microscope it opens my eyes to different but equally false unexplored dimensions.

In 1972, after house jobs, I took a *wanderjahre* and ended up at La Salpetrière hospital close to the Jardin des Plantes, where as a part of my training I was taught the value of intuition and instinctive deduction in clinical decision-making. The French neurologists who taught me were even more picturesque, more colourful in speech, manners and dress than those who had impressed me so much during my undergraduate training at The London Hospital. Symptoms were the cries of a suffering brain, and through their intense study an idea of their cause could be reached. The words for the clinical phenomena I witnessed on the wards defied accurate translation into English.

Careful observation of the external pathology was followed by a search for a physiological explanation. If this approach was not observed the image of the illness would become distorted and the patient lost from view. Jean-Martin Charcot, the father of neurology, taught me that nervous disease was very old and immutable. It was only I who would change as I learned to recognise what was formerly imperceptible. I discovered that even the classic nervous diseases like *'maladie de Parkinson'* exhibited great diversity in their course, which seemed to render them less implacable. I was acquiring a feel for sickness and an appreciation of its intricacy.

Much later I came across a footnote from William Burroughs in *Ghost of Chance* that seemed to come straight from the Leçons du Mardi:

As any astute physician well knows the progress of disease to the classic symptoms is more the exception than the rule. Any combination of the expected symptoms may be observed, or any corresponding lack of them.

The healing powers of L-DOPA had already pushed me in the direction of neurology but it was my experience at La Salpetrière in Paris that finally sealed my destiny. I seemed to be surrounded by the legendary ghosts of Joseph Babinski, Georges Gilles de la Tourette and Pierre Marie and yet some, like Charcot, still seemed to be alive.

On my return to England in 1974, I started to attend the clinical demonstrations at the National Hospital, Queen Square. Many of the famous names of British neurology taught there on Wednesday afternoons at 4 p.m. and Saturday morning at 10 a.m. to a rapt and incredulous audience. During these séances, silver-tongued senior students led us on a magical journey of inquiry. Some of these great men embellished their teaching with flourishes of showmanship but this was always backed up by a sound knowledge of semiotics. They condensed neurological mysteries into a problem and solution format and provided succinct statements of principle that provided us with a foolproof diagnostic approach that worked well in practice. Most taught off the hoof with no knowledge of the provisional diagnosis. On one occasion a man who had sustained a head injury and could only see half of everything was presented. The registrar then went on to demonstrate the half-field defect before his chief put the patient's ability to name objects to the test.

'What's this?' he asked, showing the man a half a crown. Quick as a flash and to gales of laughter the man replied 'One and threepence'.

When I began my specialist training on ward 5.2 at University College Hospital in the attic of the Cruciform building on Gower Street, British neurology was still a closed shop, with only 370 consultant posts in the whole of the British Isles. It was a highly competitive male-dominated 'boutique' speciality and the physicians at The National Hospital still exerted a strong influence on new hospital appointments and standards of good clinical practice throughout the land. Neurological apprenticeship could be compared in length and stringency to that required of a vestal virgin in Ancient Rome. Collective nouns used to describe neurologists included, 'a synapse', 'a battery' and 'a twitch' but the one I liked best was 'a galaxy'. Many of the founding fathers of London neurology had gained knighthoods and Fellowships of the Royal Society and some had unassailable names like Sir Henry Head and Lord Brain.

Nerve specialists were considered cerebral, remote and austere by their peers but in an era before non-invasive brain imaging few physicians had the knowledge or competence to question their final diagnosis. Neurologists were thinkers not doers. Jokes about their obsessionality, bow tie elegance, left-handedness and emotional coldness were common. Psychiatrists were their polar opposites and it seemed to me that their approach to medicine reflected this difference in personality. Psychiatry was woolly, dialectic and lacked physiological solidity.

Neither of my two first bosses at University College Hospital, William Gooddy and Gerald Stern, fitted the conventional image of a neurologist but they did not deviate in their approach from the diagnostic technique laid down by Jean-Martin Charcot in Paris, Moritz Romberg in Berlin and William Gowers at The National Hospital, Queen Square. They reminded me on ward rounds that searching for meaning in the stories of the neurologically ill was the only way to master neurology and that I must study my patients seriously. The intricacy of neurological and psychiatric presentations defied formulaic methodology and could never be reduced to guidelines and algorithms or defined by radiological pixels. A successful outcome to a case often turned on an ability to identify clues missed by others.

Both Dr Gooddy and Dr Stern were impressive, confident, communicated sensitively and were unhurried in their demeanour. They would begin a medical consultation by asking the patient to describe the presenting symptoms, observing carefully while they took heed of what they were being told. From time to time they would write in the notes the exact words used by the patient to describe a particular complaint. They would never interrupt but when the history had been given they would clarify points with a few carefully chosen, non-leading questions. I watched with interest how they paid particular attention to irrelevant trifles and inconsequentialities. They took notice of negatives and had an uncanny ability to expose inconsistencies. After they had satisfied themselves there was no more helpful information to be obtained from the patient they would then approach the relatives to get their side of the story. Finally they might turn to me and ask for additional details about the family history, the social situation of the patient and a summary of the abnormal findings discovered on physical examination. Before concluding their investigation they would verify at the bedside one or two physical signs where there was doubt over the interpretation or which didn't seem to fit with the rest of the clinical picture. At the end of it all they would turn courteously to the patient and explain that the team were going off to have a discussion about what to do next.

The firm then trooped off to the day room for a coffee and a plate of Bourbon biscuits prepared by the sister on Ward 5.2. Dr Gooddy and Dr Stern never trusted to general impressions and constantly stressed the importance of careful observation and accurate recording of the case history. Every gesture, every inflection of speech, every reflex, every sensory deficit was important if one was to reduce fatal error. In a deductive process that seemed to me like thinking aloud, my teachers would then locate the site of the nerve damage, and from the details of the narrative propose the likely cause for each patients' symptoms. Last of all they would attempt to establish links between the findings at the bedside and the laboratory and radiological results. When all the data was in, a firm conclusion was drawn but I was made aware of the importance of keeping an eye open for incongruities that might subsequently negate the diagnosis.

This systematic routine, passed down from one generation of neurologists to the next, had helped to save countless patients from invasive and potentially life-threatening investigations and inappropriate treatment. When we had all had our say, my chiefs would go back and talk to the patient often alone or accompanied just by the house physician. The prognosis would be imparted and the treatment plan carefully explained.

Perfection of this methodical and time-consuming approach is essential to becoming a good neurologist and I spent many hours on the wards and in the outpatient clinic trying to hone my skills. I got to grips with the complexities of the neurological examination and gained competence in the use of the ophthalmoscope, tendon hammer, tuning fork and two point discriminator. The feeling finger became another form of observation independent of eyesight. I paid attention to trivia and held on to things that made no sense.

My teachers helped me come to terms with the tension I felt when confronted with diagnostic dilemmas. They emphasised that I should only fully accept what I had read or heard after I had verified it myself. I learned most from my mistakes, and David Perkin, my senior registrar, was a great comforter when I needed to unburden my insecurities. Neurology had, and still has, more than its fair share of devastating, incurable maladies, and from time to time my teachers would curb my fondness for new discovery by reminding me of the importance of the laying on of hands and kind words. We behaved as if death was a malady from which one always recovers but I did learn to tell the painful truth without frightening people.

William Gooddy's advice to me at the end of my second teaching round came straight from the great physician William Osler. To study the phenomena of neurological disease without books was to sail an uncharted sea, but to study books without patients was not to go to sea at all. The only way to learn was by seeing and talking to patients. His recommended reading list was eccentric. He advised me to read two books: *The Complete Works of Sherlock Holmes*, described by its author Arthur Conan Doyle as 'the fairy kingdom of romance', and Marcel Proust's *À la Recherche du Temps Perdu*. Much later I realized it had been his clever way of introducing a young man embarking on his specialist training to the methods of his predecessor, William Gowers, arguably the greatest clinical neurologist that ever lived. Gooddy believed, as I do now, that in order to master a new profession the mind of the apprentice has to pass through all the stages that the art itself has displayed in its historical evolution.

The Baker Street sleuth's method of crime detection

soon proved of far greater value than anything I had read in Lord Brain's *Diseases of the Nervous System*. Each time I took the clinical history from a patient I remembered Holmes's words to John Openshaw in *The Five Orange Pips*: 'Pray give us the essential facts from the commencement and I can afterwards question you as to those details which seem to me to be most important'.

Detective work had become a metaphor for diagnostic acumen and the mysteries that exercised Sherlock Holmes shared some of the rhythms of neurological practice.

One day I had planned to teach the second year clinical medical students on a young African boy with myasthenia gravis, a disorder that leads to profound weakness of speech, difficulties in swallowing and a droopy face. Unfortunately, despite asking the nursing staff to make sure 'Mr S' did not leave the ward, when we arrived at his bed he was nowhere to be found. Undeterred, and anxious to show off my newly acquired skills, I asked the bemused group to tell me what they could deduce about the patient. The crime scene contained a spirometer, an instrument used to measure lung capacity, an eye patch and a large number of personal possessions including some comic books. After I had listened to their suggestions it seemed reasonable for me to submit, on the basis of the evidence, that the patient was young, had double vision and shortness of breath and had been in the ward for some time to undergo some form of acute treatment. The combination of respiratory problems and diplopia in a young person pointed strongly to a primary disorder of the muscles or the junction between the muscles and nerves. Holmes used a process of abductive reasoning to solve crimes and I was now incorporating this into my clinical method:

Let me see if I can make it clearer. Most people, if you describe a train of events to them, will tell you what the result would be. They can put those events together in their minds, and argue from them that something will come to pass. There are few people, however, who, if you told them a result, would be able to evolve from their own inner consciousness what the steps were which led up to that result. This power is what I mean when I talk of reasoning backward, or analytically.

– *A Study in Scarlet*

Just as we were about to leave the ward, 'Mr S' returned to his room and I was able to elicit for the students the fatiguable weakness of his eye muscles and droopiness of his eyelids, his nasal speech and mild weakness of his arms and legs compatible with the diagnosis of myasthenia gravis.

Conan Doyle knew about recent advances in the understanding of nervous diseases from his own postgraduate medical research on tabes dorsalis (one of the three common types of neurosyphilis).

In *The Adventure of the Resident Patient*, Holmes

and Watson meet a character called Dr Trevelyan, the author of 'a monograph on obscure nervous lesions'. Trevelyan tells Holmes of his interest in the study of neurology:

My own hobby has always been nervous disease. I should wish to make it an absolute speciality, but, of course a man must take what he can get.

Trevelyan had found himself in the midst of a criminal gang's feud and been asked to see a 'Russian nobleman' who had presented with catalepsy. Judging from the accurate nature of the clinical description it is likely that Conan Doyle had consulted the chapter relating to trance in William Gowers' *Manual of Diseases of the Nervous System*. Holmes quickly realises the patient is malingering and solves the case to the astonishment of Trevelyan.

To seek out clues and make rational conclusions based on findings at the bedside gave rise in me to strong feelings of satisfaction. I was also learning to build my life within the confines of the hospital. As I became more familiar with the Sherlock Holmes canon I found vignettes of St Vitus's dance, cerebral apoplexy, tetanus, delirium and meningitis that confirmed my growing suspicions that the real neurologist manqué was Sir Arthur Conan Doyle. I was enjoying the intellectual challenge of neurology and had acquired the necessary inurement to avoid being destroyed by the everyday tragedies I witnessed on the wards. The bedside was now my laboratory.

The biographies of several of the neurologists who were practising at the turn of the twentieth century shared many of the character traits of Sherlock Holmes: aloofness, panache, an air of intellectual superiority bordering on arrogance and more than a hint of misogyny. Holmes was a much greater artistic creation than the stories in which he appeared.

As my training in neurology continued at The Middlesex Hospital many of the words of advice I was learning from my new teachers Michael Kremer, Christopher Earl, Roger Gilliatt and Michael Harrison, evoked Holmes' pithy aphorisms:

One should always look for a possible alternative and provide against it. It is the first rule of criminal investigation.
    – *The Adventure of Black Peter*

Singularity is almost invariably a clue. The more featureless and commonplace a crime is, the more difficult it is to bring home.
    – *The Boscombe Valley Mystery*

You see, but you do not observe. The distinction is clear .
    – *A Scandal in Bohemia*

I never guess. It is a shocking habit – destructive to the logical faculty.
    – *The Sign of Four*

How often have I said to you that when you have eliminated the impossible, whatever remains, however improbable, must be the truth?

– *The Sign of Four*

They were teaching me to focus like Holmes on the rubbish heap of despised and unnoticed observations.

In the 1970s, neurology in Great Britain was a very competitive and oversubscribed speciality and I felt honoured to have been given a chance to throw my hat in the ring. I had the great privilege of coming into contact with chiefs who were inspirational, generous, understanding and helpful. Most of my teachers at both University College Hospital and the Middlesex Hospital felt as uncomfortable as I did about an elitist system that denied women full and equal employment opportunities. I now knew that the wisdom I had learned from textbooks and lectures would never give me the knowledge of when to probe and when to leave alone, when to reassure and when to keep silent. Gowers' nineteenth-century writings were different. They read like novels and brought the diseases I was now studying to life. I also knew that, however sophisticated technology became, it could never be a substitute for taking a detailed history. Patients were my main teachers. They could not be reduced to a repository of deranged regulatory systems or a collection of malfunctioning organs. Benway's descriptions of his brain-damaged patients at the Freeland Reconditioning Centre were no longer funny but preposterous:

'Come and take a close look,' says Benway. 'You won't embarrass anybody'. I walk over and stand in front of a man who is sitting on his bed. I look at the man's eyes. Nobody, nothing looks back. 'IND's', says Benway, 'Irreversible Neural Damage. Overliberated you might say . . . a drag on the industry'. I pass a hand in front of the man's eyes. 'Yes,' says Benway,'they still have reflexes. Watch this'. Benway takes a chocolate bar from his pocket, removes the wrapper and holds it in front of the man's nose. The man sniffs. His jaws begin to work. He makes snatching motions with his hands. Saliva drips from his mouth and hangs off his chin in long streamers.
– *Naked Lunch*

My future was still uncertain but I had managed to curb my contrariness and obduracy. I loved the reasoning involved in diagnosis and as my competence improved I was able to relax, become less defensive and be more responsive to my patients' despair. I tried to acquire the habit of entering into the feelings of my patients and into their modes of thought. I had come to realise that the lives of the neurologically ill were far more richly detailed and sensational than their misfortune suggested. Their colourful, spirited and often painful stories gave me insight into how I could ease their suffering. Listening attentively to the narrative from which my patients came and to which – well or ill – they were bound to return, held the key. Stories were what provided all of us with an identity for the place we lived in and for ourselves as individuals. Clinical judgement was a vital counterpoise to the rationality of science with its calculations, impartiality and disinterestedness. As I got better at 'whodunit' I also began to search for answers as to why the crime had been committed in the first place. I started to understand that neurology began where Doctor Watson always did: with the circumstances of the case.

William Burroughs had returned to America in 1974, in the same year Richard Nixon became the first American President forced to resign from office. Burroughs was now famous and acclaimed as an important writer but he was still on the run from 'the ugly spirit'. I had now read his memoir *Junkie: Confessions of an Unredeemed Drug Addict*, *The Yage Letters*, *Interzone* and *The Ticket that Exploded* but could not relate any of these books to my work as a hospital doctor.

After graduation from Harvard, Burroughs toyed briefly with a career in psychiatry but within a few months of enrolling for a medical degree in Vienna in 1936, he had concluded that despite the amenability of the medical profession to accommodate individuals of widely differing character, he was totally unsuitable for the profession:

I could never have been a doctor. I did right to quit. My heart

is too soft and too hard, too quickly moved to love, anger or
indifference. I would care too much for some patients and
nothing for others.

– *Interzone*

One connection that intrigued me was the discovery that his Columbia University friends Allen
Ginsberg, Jack Kerouac and Edie Parker had all likened 'Old Bull Lee' (Burroughs) to a real-life Sherlock
Holmes. Burroughs was something of a dandy in the
grand English tradition, always courteous and impeccably dressed in Saville Row suits. He smoked Senior
Service cigarettes, ate at Rules and shopped at Fortnum
and Mason. In the 1940s he had worked as a private eye,
hoping to enter the noir world of Dashiell Hammett,
but had been disappointed with the triviality of the
case material. Like Holmes he had resorted to cocaine
as a cure for ennui usually in the form of 'speedballs'
and he kept a firearm under his pillow. There was also
a physical resemblance: Burroughs was tall with cold
piercing eyes, an aquiline nose and thin lips.

Ever since his time at university, Burroughs had developed the habit of retreating to his room for days on
end. He was a master of disguise and shared the fictional detective's strong antipathy to women and nuanced
sexuality. Both were outsiders and anti-authoritarian.
But there were obvious differences too. Burroughs
was peripatetic, addicted to narcotics and more anar-
chic. Holmes preferred chemistry whereas Burroughs'

forensic investigations embraced telepathy and extra-sensory perception. I now saw Burroughs more as a freelance investigator researching anthropology, psychology, biology, sociology and neuroscience in an attempt to accurately inform his fiction:

... after I got out of Harvard in 1936, I had done some graduate work in anthropology. I got a glimpse of academic life and didn't like it at all. It looked like there was too much faculty intrigue, faculty teas, cultivating the head of the department so on and so forth.

– *Paris Review* interview with Conrad Knickerbocker in St Louis, 1965

Just as things seemed to be progressing well in my career and I had started to relish medical life I read an article that had first appeared in the May 1974 issue of *The Lancet.* It was entitled *Medical Nemesis,* written by a Catholic priest called Ivan Illich. It began with the unsettling words:

Within the last decade medical professional practice has become a major threat to health. Depression, infection, disability, dysfunction, and other specific iatrogenic diseases now cause more suffering than all accidents from traffic or industry. Beyond this, medical practice sponsors sickness by the reinforcement of a morbid society, which not only industrially preserves its defectives but breeds the therapist's client in a cybernetic way. Finally, the so-called health-professions have an indirect sickening power – a structurally health-denying effect.

Illich believed the medical profession were on a fruitless mission to eradicate pain, sickness and even death and was doing a great deal of harm by whipping up unrealistic expectations. Old age, handicap and death had been handed over by society to doctors to keep families from having to face them:

Doctors deploy themselves as they like, more so than other professionals, and they tend to gather where the climate is healthy, where the water is clean, and where people are employed and can pay for their services.

Illich warned of disease caused as a direct consequence of medical and surgical intervention:

A culture can become prey of a pharmaceutical invasion. Each culture has its poisons, its remedies, its placebos, and its ritual settings for their administration. Most of these are destined for the healthy rather than the sick.

Doctors had become the high priests of 'a vast monolithic religion' and the teaching hospital was geared for them rather than their patients. They had entered into a Faustian bargain that replaced healing with treatment, listening with investigations and caring with managing. The distressed human was divorced from the transaction.

Illich's doomsday prediction did not seem to have reached the National Health Service yet but it was a severe warning that I knew could easily come true. I wondered what Burroughs was thinking as he read Illich's writings in his dark windowless room at 222 The Bowery ('The Bunker'). He had written that schools should teach values, not facts, and shared many of Illich's views about the shortcomings of modern medicine and the rottenness of Western Society. He also warned that technological advances could be highly dangerous in the wrong hands. He would have rejected Illich's vicarious tolerance of pain even if he accepted his imputations of conspiracy by those who were paid to relieve it. Unlike Illich, Burroughs was not against painless dentistry, the use of modern antibiotics and anaesthesia.

In the end my fascination with neurology prevailed. I pushed Illich and his uncomfortable views to the back of my brain and returned to the pleasure of listening to patients' stories in the clinics.

5

– Hanging Out with the Molecules –

Many of the patients I was now seeing in the research clinic at University College Hospital had started to worry that they were becoming allergic or resistant to their drugs. They complained that some doses of L-DOPA, especially when taken with large meals, failed to work and that they could no longer rely on four or five hours benefit from each tablet. When their pill came on-stream it was as if someone had switched the light back on but they were having more and more Cinderella moments of disablement. Flinging helicopter movements of the limbs and distressing involuntary grimaces marred their sense of well-being even during their shrinking periods of mobility. One told me he now knew where the Monty Python Ministry of Silly Walks had come from. Another felt as if he was on a tightrope. The patients described tingling and stiffening followed by a terrifying sensation of their batteries running down. Some reported visions of motionless, silent Lilliputians and shadowy presences. Others had hallucinations of animals sitting in their homes or stalking the garden and grey mice scuttling across the floor.

'DB', a teacher who had developed Parkinson's

disease at the age of thirty-six, arrived in a wheelchair in great pain from contortions of his arms and legs to tell me tearfully that life with L-DOPA had come to resemble a never-ending big dipper ride. When he left the outpatient clinic twenty minutes later 'cured' and walking briskly, my reputation as a healer was greatly enhanced with the receptionists but all that had happened was that his medication had lit up his dopamine brain during the consultation. These were erratic 'all or none' occurrences. Everything was capricious. Nothing was predictable.

I felt I was on a voyage of discovery and that if I could record and document accurately what I was now seeing I might be able to decipher a chaos that appeared to defy the laws of pharmacology. I began to think it was amazing that L-DOPA had ever worked in the first place. I also now accepted that making an individual whole again couldn't be reduced to the prescription of a treatment however effective it was in improving quality of life. The art of medicine was not to be confused with artfulness. It had nothing to do with smoke and mirrors but was a skill born out of experience and practice and a knowledge of universals.

Clinical pharmacology was a great strength at University College when I arrived in 1974. James Black, Nobel Laureate who had developed propranolol for the control of angina pectoris and cimetidine for the treatment of peptic ulceration, had moved from his post in industry to establish a new degree course in medicinal chemistry. Desmond Laurence, Professor of Clinical Pharmacology at University College Hospital, had written the definitive undergraduate textbook on his subject and was an inspiring presence at the Clinical Grand Rounds. As young doctors in training we were encouraged to test new drugs on ourselves and on patient volunteers in the wards.

Not long after I had begun my specialist neurology training at University College Hospital, the head of the medical department at Sandoz approached my chief, Gerald Stern, with an offer to test a new molecule in the clinic. The new drug 2-brom-alpha-ergocriptine (bromocriptine), synthesised from the naturally occurring alkaloid ergocryptine, was a potent stimulator of brain dopamine receptors and a candidate anti-Parkinson drug. Although the Sandoz Company had been forced to discontinue the sale of LSD-25 (Delysid) in 1965 it had maintained a research interest in the medicinal potential of ergot compounds obtained from the rye fungus (*Claviceps purpurea*) and ergotamine was still in use for the treatment of acute migraine while ergometrine was used by obstetricians to expel the afterbirth.

After we had obtained ethical approval I began to cautiously escalate the dose of bromocriptine in ten patients who had either been recently diagnosed with Parkinson's disease or who had been unable to tolerate L-DOPA treatment. At doses above 40 mg a day their symptoms of slowness, stiffness and trembling started to lessen to a level that could be appreciated without the need to consult the rating scales I was using to give my study a pseudo-scientific robustness.

These preliminary findings that were published in the 14 October 1975 issue of *The Lancet* encouraged me to use bromocriptine in more previously untreated patients with Parkinson's disease in the hope that the drug might avoid some of the complications that were now occurring commonly in the clinic with L-DOPA. I also started to look for groups of patients with related parkinsonian disorders that had been unable to tolerate or had not responded to standard drug therapy.

A few of the survivors of the pandemic of sleepy sickness were still living in the villas of the Highlands Hospital (previously the Northern Convalescent Fever Hospital), just north of Winchmore Hill in Enfield, where a special long stay unit for 100 children aged between three and sixteen had been established in 1925. Most of them had developed a unique neuropsychiatric syndrome that resembled Parkinson's disease but differed in its presentation, course and response to medication.

The surviving Highlands Hospital postencephalitics had been given a one-month trial of L-DOPA in 1969. After less than two weeks of treatment, pathological imbalances of the sort that I was only now starting to see in the patients with Parkinson's disease at University College Hospital had emerged in several of the patients. Ten had experienced wild jerky twisting movements of their tongue, lips, face and limbs, six had become mentally agitated and manic, two had complained of shortness of breath and one woman had developed severe anxiousness with constant high-pitched moaning. Unfortunately, the severity of damage to the dopamine-containing nerve cells in their brains had rendered them exquisitely sensitive to the treatment and only two out of the forty had derived lasting, useful benefit from L-DOPA for more than a year. They were ideal candidates for the bromocriptine trial.

Encephalitis lethargica (sleepy sickness) is a virus of the mind that causes a kaleidoscope of bizarre and bewildering neurological and psychiatric symptoms. About five million people fell prey to the disease between 1916 and 1927, many of whom died. The brunt of the damage occurs in the 'lizard brain,' inherited from our pre-mammalian forebears and a sanctum for the interplay of motion and emotion. Impulsive, obsessional and enraged behaviours are common sequelae. The plague allowed tics and antics to mushroom in the dark cellars of the basal ganglia, nurtured by spurts of dopamine.

During his time working at Beth Abraham Hospital in the Bronx, Doctor Oliver Sacks wrote several letters to *The Lancet* describing the effects of L-DOPA on the signs of parkinsonism in a similar postencephalitic colony. Under pressure from his medical director, who saw little point in adding to the correspondence section of a British medical journal, he was then browbeaten to write up his overall experience in sixty patients for the *Journal of the American Medical Association*. His article in the September 1970 issue drew particular attention to the hazardous reactions to the drug and the emergence of a phenomenon he referred to as incontinent nostalgia. The startling physical and mental rebirths of the patients had been followed by retribution and finally a painful re-adjustment and accommodation to their imprisonment.

The entire correspondence in the letters section of the next edition was devoted to highly critical and bitter responses to his article, questioning his accuracy of observation and intimating that even if true he should have thought hard before publishing the findings because it would negatively impact on the atmosphere of optimism necessary for a positive L-DOPA response. The editor permitted no right of reply. Sacks' article had cast doubt on predictability itself and needed to be censored. Rational discussion was scarcely possible. Much more distressing though was when the sister of Rose R., one of his patients, held up the *New York Daily News* that had reprinted word for word one of Sacks' letters to *The Lancet*, complaining, 'Is this your medical discretion?'

Sacks now felt trapped. He knew he had something of importance to say but if he were to remain faithful to his experiences he would inevitably forfeit medical 'publishability' and the acceptance of his colleagues. He would be at risk of losing the serious stamp of science. If he were to write the detailed case histories of his patients, he would also need to obtain their unconditional consent and disguise their identity and the institution involved. His friend, W. H. Auden, gave him particularly good advice in the planning phase for the intended book. 'You're going to have to go beyond the clinical . . . Be metaphorical, be mystical, be whatever you need.'

When *Awakenings* was published in 1973 it was reviewed positively in the newspapers and by the literary magazines and awarded the Hawthornden Prize for imaginative literature. Sacks had taken Auden's advice and attacked the mechanical methodologies insisted upon by medical journals and epitomised by the early reports of L-DOPA in Parkinson's disease that he described as 'the ugliest exemplars of assembly-line medicine; everything human, everything living, pounded, ground, pulverized, atomized, quantized, and otherwise "processed" out of existence'.

However, a strange silence lasting more than a year prevailed in most of the medical press before a few short and mixed reviews trickled out. Sacks found one particularly galling:

This is an amazing book, the more so since Sacks is talking about non-existent patients in a non-existent hospital, patients with a non-existent disease, because there was no worldwide epidemic of sleepy sickness in the 1920s.

– *On the Move: A Life*

I did not meet Oliver Sacks for several more years but his experience following the publication of *Awakenings* provided me with a salutary reminder of the conservatism of the medical establishment. Doctor Sacks had crossed the line and was now considered an eccentric.

With the help of Dr Joseph Sharkey, the Medical Director, I selected twelve of the most severely handicapped patients who had been inmates in the Highlands Hospital for more than half a century, and despite their negative experiences with L-DOPA they were still game to try another experimental drug. I felt it a great privilege to be allowed into this secret world that seemed to be suspended in time. For the next year, this out of the way hospital would become the home for my scientific experiments. One of the trial volunteers had been nicknamed Puskás by the nurses after the Hungarian football maestro of the 1950s. For most of the last forty-five years he had remained catatonic, barely able to move, and in need of help for all everyday tasks. However, when one of the nurses threw him a ball, he sprang to life, trapping the ball adroitly with his feet and dribbling skilfully down the ward. He could also juggle a matchbox on one foot, kick it in the air, catch it in his hand, drop it to the floor and kick it up again. On one occasion I watched him use this sensory trick to allow him to hop the length of the ward. If a fly landed on his nose he was able to whisk it away smartly with his hand.

Another of the postencephalitics had for many years shared a room with a fellow sufferer of similar age in the 12A pavilion. Both showed little interest in their surroundings and were mute. One day a loud noise came from the usually silent room and on entering I found that the two living statues had come alive and were wrestling one another and bellowing insults. As soon as they were separated, they froze up again and remained inert on all my subsequent visits. I had witnessed my first examples of a phenomenon called *Kinesia paradoxica* that had allowed chairbound postencephalitics to run to escape house fires and earthquakes or swim to safety from a sinking ship. If I could understand better this natural unblocking mechanism and how to trigger it, a new drug treatment for Parkinson's disease might become unnecessary.

Some of the survivors at Highlands also had strange speech disturbances. Every time I questioned one woman she involuntarily repeated a meaningless phrase over and over again. When I then asked her to recite the Lord's Prayer, she did so fluently with no trace of hesitation or repetition. Another patient echoed everything that was said to him. One of the elderly charge nurses told me that many years ago there was another lady who rarely spoke but would bellow foul obscenities for no apparent reason. These patients made me think about Burroughs' view that language was an affliction, an alien organism that hi-jacked the perceptions of its unsuspecting host:

From symbiosis to parasitism is a short step. The word is now a virus. The flu virus may have once been a healthy lung cell. It is now a parasitic organism that invades and damages the central nervous system. Modern man has lost the option of silence. Try halting sub-vocal speech. Try to achieve even ten seconds of inner silence. You will encounter a resisting organism that forces you to talk. That organism is the word.

– *The Ticket that Exploded*

Did these patients that had remained tight-lipped for so long continue to listen to stillness and communicate internally above the din? As Burroughs had said 'the most addictive drug of all is silence'.

I longed to release the brakes from these forgotten patients and bring them back to the land of the living. After I had got to know them and recorded their level of handicap, I started the trial drug in low doses. Each week, on my half day of study leave from University College Hospital, I travelled by bus to Southgate and walked down World's End Lane. Although now an acute general hospital with five hundred beds, Highlands still had the look of an isolated concentration camp with a gothic central administration block, sinister chimney stacks and a winding lane of two storey L-shaped red and yellow brick buildings with coved eaves. Every time I entered pavilion 12A, my hopes of seeing improvement on the increased dose of bromo-criptine were dashed. The drug was better tolerated than L-DOPA but its therapeutic effect on Puskás and the other volunteers was deeply disappointing.

Although the clinical features of some of the postencephalitics closely resembled those seen in Par-kinson's disease, the extent and severity of damage that had occurred deep in their brains meant that although they still had the capacity to respond to dopamine replacement, their response to drugs was far more ex-treme and unpredictable. The landscapes in which the postencephalitics resided were far bleaker than people with Parkinson's disease.

Meanwhile, a few of the group of previously untreated patients at University College Hospital, who had ben-efited for more than a year from large doses of bromo-criptine, had started to run into difficulties. One day I was rung up by the duty psychiatric registrar to inform me that a woman who I knew well had been admitted to the North Wing at St Pancras Hospital with ideas of persecution. When I went to visit her, she spoke to me in a highly pressured uncharacteristic fashion and complained that the authorities wanted her back at University College Hospital 'dead or alive'. She in-formed me that the doctors were 'trying to change her mind' and that the nurses had poisoned her food.

As I moved to sit at the end of the bed, she became

agitated in case I squashed a Siamese cat asleep on the cover. One thing that interested me as we talked was that despite her delirium, her signs of Parkinson's disease seemed much less. I suggested to the psychiatrists that her bromocriptine be reduced down to 30 mg a day and that she continue with the mild tranquillisers they had prescribed for at least two more weeks. Within 48 hours her delusions settled, and the distressing hallucinations that had included a number of faceless men sitting in chairs had vanished. When I saw her in the clinic at University College Hospital, she told me that during her time in the North Wing she had seen flowing visions of enhanced colour and had felt as if time had stopped still for the days of her admission. She was now back to her usual lucid self but her greatly improved mobility that I had witnessed while she was confused had now disappeared and she was again scuffing her soles and not swinging her arms when she walked.

A few months later, another of the volunteers from the bromocriptine trial returned to clinic complaining of burning in the fingers and toes and severe cramping in her calves when walking that forced her to pull up and rest after about a hundred metres. On examination she was disorientated, had deathly white hands and an ashen nose. The normal pulsations in the arteries of her feet were impalpable and her radial pulse was thready. Her symptoms resembled those first described in the seventeenth-century epidemics

of St Anthony's Fire, caused by eating rye bread contaminated with *Claviceps purpurea* fungus. No cases of
ergotism caused by bromocriptine had been reported,
but I felt nevertheless that this was the likely diagnosis.
I stopped the trial drug at once and switched her over
to L-DOPA; she recovered completely over the next
four weeks and gangrene was avoided.

The following week I took a call from the worried son of Mrs N, an elderly lady who had worked as
a cleaner all her life and been diagnosed three years
earlier with Parkinson's disease. He told me that his
mother had started to compulsively squander all her
pension money on bingo and he had begun to wonder
whether the bromocriptine she was taking had anything to do with it. I told him I was not aware of any
link between gambling and the new drug but to contact me again if things deteriorated. My own view was
that his mother was probably very lonely and it was her
way of trying to cheer herself up.

Things got much worse and Mrs N's son made an
emergency appointment for her to see me. He told me
she was now visiting the bingo hall four days a week
and had fallen behind with her rent. Although his
mother vehemently denied intemperate gambling, he
estimated that she had lost several thousand pounds
in the last few months. It was hard to know who was
telling the truth. After excusing myself, I stepped out
of the clinic room and called the Medical Information Department at Sandoz, whereupon I was told that

two cases of pathological gambling had already been reported with bromocriptine but a clear and definite cause and effect had not been established. To the son's relief, I tapered down his mother's bromocriptine and when she returned to clinic six weeks later, she told me that she had given up bingo altogether.

The most exciting finding to come out of my continuing work with bromocriptine was that when the drug was used alone to treat the symptoms of Parkinson's disease, it provided sustained symptom relief without the volleys of jolting twitches and convulsive movements seen with L-DOPA. Considered at best a long shot, bromocriptine had far exceeded expectations and been shown to be a very effective treatment for Parkinson's disease. However, it was also now clear the medicine carried a considerable risk, and doubts were being expressed on whether it was safe for routine use. This vicissitude in bromocriptine's fortune replicated the twists and turns in the path to acceptance of most effective treatments. New drugs were often the subject of exaggeratedly enthusiastic accolades, followed by excessively critical reappraisal. Clinical experience usually showed that the truth lay somewhere in the middle and eventually, despite concerns about its unwanted psychiatric side effects, bromocriptine became a popular medicine with many experts recommending it as first line treatment in younger patients with Parkinson's disease.

Albert Hofmann, a former director of medical

research at Sandoz, had shown that all the naturally occurring alkaloids extracted from the rye fungus *Claviceps purpurea* were derived from a single building block. Substitutions in the tetracyclic indole ring of lysergic acid determined the type and action of each of the naturally occurring ergot alkaloids.

One day, Hofmann was dabbling with this basic structure in the hope of developing a new powerful analeptic when he isolated d-lysergic acid diethylamide (LSD). The drug did not seem a promising candidate for therapeutic trials as it caused unsteadiness and catatonia in animals. He put the unusually fragile molecule to one side. A few years later, he synthesised a new batch of LSD and decided to re-investigate its properties. During the course of one experiment, he was overcome by a pleasant and unexpected state of intoxication. On getting home, he closed his eyes and was treated to an uninterrupted, two-hour stream of extraordinary pictures and astonishing geometric shapes. He concluded correctly that he must have inhaled or ingested a very small dose of LSD. A few days later, he deliberately took what he imagined to be the tiny dose of 250 micrograms. He immediately felt terrified and giddy and asked his laboratory assistant to accompany him home by bicycle. On the way home, he noticed that the sound of cars was transformed into optical effects and colours changed rapidly from one radiant hue to another. All the effects wore off after six hours. Hoffmann had written himself into the annals of psychedelia by taking the first ever recorded acid trip.

Publication of his results caused a sensation. It was hoped that LSD-25, 'the medicine of the soul', could help shed light on the biology of schizophrenia and other serious mental disorders. Sandoz introduced the drug commercially in 1947. The CIA began a research programme that involved administering it without informed consent to military personnel, government agents and prostitutes. In the sixties, Timothy Leary, a Harvard academic, suggested the drug could induce a heavenly sunlit inner quietude and provide a better treatment for the mentally ill. Leary considered the brain to be a biochemical electrical network capable of creating a changing series of adaptive realities. He wrote that the language of God was not English or Latin but cellular and molecular.

Leary went to Tangier in July 1961 to meet Burroughs and invited him to visit his Centre for Research in Personality. In a letter written from Harvard the previous January, Leary had described the political situation as far as psychedelic drugs were concerned:

Medicine has already pre-empted LSD, marijuana is the football for two other powerful groups – Bohemia and the narcotics agents. Mescaline and psilocybin are still up for grabs and it is our hope to keep them ungrabbed, uncontrolled, available.

– *Rub out the Words*

On his return to the International Zone of Tangier, Burroughs told his literary friend, Paul Bowles, that 'Doctor Tim' had the most unscientific mind he had ever encountered and that he did not condone Leary's proselytizing of psychedelic drugs for personal development. Despite his distaste for scientists, Burroughs never equated a scientific paper with a piece of imaginative poetry. After a rocky start, Burroughs and Leary got on fine and shared the view that the only hope for the world lay in exploration of the galaxies and the development of space colonies.

In England, during my medical student days, Timothy Leary was portrayed in the tabloid press as a disgraced lunatic, but for hippies during the Summer of Love he was considered a visionary. When asked about Burroughs in a 1989 interview for *Pataphysics*, Leary said:

He's a very scientific person. The only psychedelic he likes is marijuana . . . Burroughs has forgotten more about drugs in his life than I've learned. Burroughs is in charge of his life. He knows what he's doing . . . But Burroughs, he's not the guy that goes around with a grin on his face saying peace and love. He's a very crusty, introverted guy with a deep sense of humour. He's one of the funniest persons alive – it's a very laid-back kind of humor.

More than 30,000 mental patients, including some with alcoholism, were treated with LSD and more than a thousand peer review papers were published between 1957 and 1967. Psychiatrists considered its main value was in facilitating the psychoanalytical process and relieving anxiety. The response to a dose of the drug, however, was highly unpredictable and some acutely psychotic patients deteriorated after treatment, with their hallucinations acquiring a menacing and phantasmagorical quality. Reports of young people 'flying' to their death after taking LSD for recreational purposes and the Manson murders, led to mounting public concern. Richard Nixon stated that Timothy Leary was 'the most dangerous man in America' and put him in jail for drugs offences. Senator Robert Kennedy on the other hand, questioned this sudden shift of opinion: 'Perhaps to some extent we have lost sight of the fact that (LSD) can be very, very helpful in our society if used properly.' In response to its increasing use by leading lights in the countercultural movement, the United States made LSD-25 illegal in 1966.

The molecule's hallucinogenic properties were thought to be due to its stimulant effects on the brain's 5-hydroxytryptamine (serotonin) receptors but, like bromocriptine, it also stimulated dopamine receptors. When I compared the structural formula of the bromocriptine molecule with that of LSD-25, I understood why some of my patients had seen cinematic visions, misidentified shapes and people, and become convinced that mice were running across the floor.

I even thought about a trial of Hofmann's 'problem

child' LSD-25 in Parkinson's disease but Burroughs' warnings about 'backbrain stimulants' held me back. In a 1966 letter to the *New Statesman*, Burroughs had written:

I can speak from experience about the hallucinogenic drugs having experimented over a period of years with LSD, mescaline, psilocybin, dimethyltryptamine. I consider these drugs more dangerous than useful. They can produce states of acute pain and anxiety even death, as occurred last year in London to a doctor who had taken a 'safe' dose. Toxic effects are more liable to occur after several exposures than on first use – that is we are dealing with a phenomena of decreased tolerance or sensitisation.

– *Rub out the Words*

Fear of censorship by my peers also restrained me but the tie-up between psychedelic drugs and Parkinson's disease was something I stored up in my brain attic for possible future scientific exploration. Medical history had taught me that something that was not specifically sought and owed nothing to hypothesis-driven research could culminate in an important discovery. I hoped that serendipity and random recombination could help me find a molecule that could permanently reset the catecholamine imbalance to the default position and loosen the rigid structures of the brain.

6

– The Speed Laboratory –

After two years in the hospital my clinical skills had improved sufficiently for me to embark on the next phase of my training. Although the chemical revolution had stalled and Parkinson's disease remained incurable, clinical pharmacology was still an exciting field. There was growing optimism that the advances taking place in the life sciences would soon translate to new treatments and in 1978 I was excited to be given an opportunity to pitch for glory in the 'serotonin lab' of Gerald Curzon at the Institute of Neurology in Chenies Mews.

I found out quickly that neurological practice and research were two different worlds with very different methodologies and incommensurate languages. Science required an appreciation of balanced experimental design. Everything had to be quantified or calculated if it was to be believed. It spoke in jargon and impenetrable prose.

My project was to inject albino Sprague-Dawley rats with a high dose of d-amphetamine and then observe how drugs with different effects on the brain's serotonin (5-hydroxytryptamine) pathways further modified the animals' behaviour. Serotonin was believed to play an important role in the regulation of appetite and sleep and low brain levels had been linked to depression.

Amphetamines release dopamine from nerve terminals. They cause rodents to rear up, sniff and lick, weave their heads from side to side and run aggressively up and down in their cages. My experiments were designed to explore serotonin's interaction with dopamine.

At a dose of 15 milligrams per kilogram of d-amphetamine, the rats circled and walked backwards. These peculiar behaviours were similar to those seen with hallucinogens including LSD-25 and mescaline in laboratory animals. They also resembled the repetitive rotations seen in caged zoo animals and the behavioural vices of disturbed farm animals. After I had quantified the individual behaviours using laboratory counters and rating scales, I would then inject one of a panel of drugs known to modify brain serotonin. One of the drugs I used was fluoxetine, which blocked the re-uptake of serotonin into the nerve terminals and would later be marketed as Prozac, the best-selling and controversial drug for depression.

At the end of each experiment, I would guillotine the rats, dissect their brain from the skull and freeze the tissue for neurochemical analysis. My naive idea of work in a laboratory had been based on the apparent infallibility of routine blood tests and the ease of ordering investigations on the wards. As I learned to centrifuge, homogenise, pipette, amplify and sacrifice in a vain attempt to acquire the tools of the trade, I realised that the skills I had learned in the hospital were of negligible use in the lab.

Although neurology training took many years and the prospect of obtaining a consultant post in a teaching hospital was small, the career path for the young doctoral scientists I now worked with was far more uncertain. Their shorter working day and relative freedom from responsibility hardly justified their risible pay scale. During my short stay in the laboratory some of my colleagues, trying to live on salaries barely above the minimum working wage, were forced to sell their souls to the pharmaceutical industry, join the brain drain or reluctantly abandon research altogether and take positions as laboratory managers or administrators. It was the Winter of Discontent and I came to see those who clung to their scientific principles as admirable idealists.

Amphetamines were first synthesised in the late nineteenth century but little interest was shown in them until the 1930s when the pharmaceutical company Smith, Kline and French introduced Benzedrine (dl-amphetamine) inhalers for the relief of hay fever and asthma. Amphetamines were also found to have mild benefits in Parkinson's disease and became established as a treatment for depression, hyperactivity and poor attention in children. During World War II they were widely used by the Allies to combat fatigue and increase bravado but concerns about the increasingly widespread use of 'Mother's little helpers' and 'Purple Hearts' in the 1960s led to their recreational ('off-label') use being outlawed in Europe and North America. It was hardly surprising that a class of drugs reported to give limitless energy, increase vigilance, aid weight loss and improve sexual performance, might prove attractive to human beings. Stockbrokers were able to stay up all night to play the international markets and be in the office the following morning fresh as daisies. Unscrupulous professional sportsmen got an edge on their adversaries, broke records and achieved a tarnished glory. Long distance truck drivers reached ever more demanding deadlines without falling asleep at the wheel. 'Speed', as it was known on the street, offered a short cut to prosperity and bliss and incited the capitalist dream. I thought of Jack Kerouac's day and night typing of *On the Road* where he had used a continuous scroll of paper to allow him to record passively each and every event over a three-week Benzedrine jag:

Benny has made me see a lot. The process of intensifying awareness naturally leads to an overflow of old notions, and voila, new material wells up like water forming its proper level, and makes itself evident at the brim of consciousness.

Kerouac claimed that amphetamines had accelerated his thought processes and allowed him to write in 'the now'. They helped him to find a new, spontaneous way of writing that banished convention and directly communicated raw physical and emotional experience. In contrast to Burroughs, who revised over and over again, Kerouac believed the first draft was always the best.

Most scientific papers were riddled with technical language and obscure acronyms and used specialised terms that made them incomprehensible to all but the cognoscenti. I learned about prejudices, conceit, jealousies, and pressure to publish and also how difficult it could be to reproduce the results even of one's own experiments. Some of the referees of my first publications seemed positively vindictive. One night, after a long day with 'the speed rats' when I was supposed to be writing up my research at home, Burroughs spoke to me – I pulled out *Junkie* and read what it was like for him to be on 'Bennys':

I began talking very fast. My mouth was dry and my spit came out in round white balls-spitting cotton, it's called. [. . .] I was full of expansive benevolent feelings and suddenly wanted to call on people I hadn't seen in months or even years, people I did not like and who did not like me.

Burroughs also wrote that the suspiciousness of many amphetamine addicts was justified because their interminable, rambling, agitated monologues alienated even their friends. I then turned to his scientific analysis that had been published in the Appendix of *Naked Lunch*:

This is a cerebral stimulant like cocaine. Large doses cause prolonged sleeplessness with feelings of exhilaration. The period of euphoria is followed by a horrible depression. The drug tends to increase anxiety. It causes indigestion and loss of appetite.

His descriptions of 'speed' stuck in my head; those I had read in standard pharmacology textbooks did not. It was his mixing of registers that was so imprinting – one minute clean and clinical and the next throwing in an unruly, inappropriate phrase. Writing up my research demanded a dry, storyless discourse governed by abstract nouns, tangled clauses and passive verbs. I needed Burroughs' colourful and authentic prose to revive me.

The circling and backward walking seen in the rats had been caused by a massive outpouring of dopamine and was increased further by serotonin release. These studies in the laboratory gave me the idea to investigate drugs that antagonised serotonin in the brain as potential treatments for the abnormal involuntary movements and visual illusions seen as complications of L-DOPA in Parkinson's disease.

After several rejections, my printed communications were eventually published. These sanitised articles didn't tell half the story but I was proud of them.

My unembroidered scientific papers were a travesty in that the experiments had all been conceived with some unacknowledged expectation of outcome. They provided a misleading narrative of the process of thought and glossed over observations considered irrelevant by my superiors. They had been composed in such a way as to deny the importance of inspired guesses. I felt then – as I still do – that the discussion section of the paper should come at the beginning and not at the end.

One unanswered question that intrigued me was why half the rats had consistently circled clockwise and the other half anticlockwise. On my first visit to the United States, I visited the laboratory of Stanley Glick, a scientist working at Mount Sinai Hospital in New York, who told me that he had got the answer. Rats, like humans, have an innate laterality bias with subtle differences in the appearance of the cerebral hemispheres and different levels of grey matter dopamine on the two sides of their brains.

Parkinson's disease typically presented with symptoms down one side of the body and there was usually a delay of at least two or three years before disabilities became apparent on the other side. The malady also remained asymmetrical through its whole course and was associated with a spinal curvature to one or other side. My time in the laboratory was almost over, and the circling amphetamine rat gradually lost favour as a test bed for investigating brain dopamine function. I felt an opportunity might have been missed to explain clinical phenomena that continued to defy adequate explanation.

There was a huge gulf between scientific research and medical practice. Science was all about induction not deduction; discovery and proof were separate activities. My colleagues in the laboratory had been kind and helpful but saw me as a well-paid dilettante, ticking a box on an alien career path. Although I was impressed by the boundless optimism and enthusiasm for exploration of some of the scientists, others came over as menial public servants restricted by government dictates and reluctant to stick their heads above the parapet. One or two seemed to gain greater pleasure from tidying up the laboratory than conducting experiments. I think they were all dismayed at my sloppiness of thinking and subjective, discursive viewpoint. On the other hand, I was astonished by their lack of understanding of the handicaps caused by neurodegenerative disease and surprised that they did not see the importance of talking to patients.

To be productive most scientists need the company of fellow researchers whose expertise complements their own, a functional laboratory, productive competition and a quiet, conventional life. Discussions over coffee had convinced me that almost all scientific research led nowhere and on the rare occasions when it did, it often kicked off in a completely different direction from where it started. Common sense was as useful in research as it was in clinical practice, and in my view there was no such thing as unprejudiced observation. The scientists I worked with swore, made mistakes and quarrelled but the good ones had honesty and integrity. Good fortune and intuition cropped up everywhere and cherry picking seemed part of the game. The Eureka moments had often come during dreams or states of intoxication. Scientists, like doctors, were of strikingly different temperaments and worked in divergent ways. Explorers, gumshoes, artists and even mystics stood tall in their ranks. Green fingers seemed as important as scrupulous scientific method in sifting a grain of fact from a mountain of fool's gold.

I was glad to have gathered an understanding of the difficulties inherent in laboratory work and the discipline needed to create order from mayhem. I had also picked up the rudiments of statistics and learned how many failures lay behind each successful experiment. I now understood that it was the criticism of gathered facts that gave science its true individuality and universalism. If in the future I was to go on to convince myself and others of something I only guessed to be true, I would need to forge lasting collaborations with open-minded and sympathetic neurobiologists who understood that patients must always be centre stage in medical research. Their rigour and ingenuity would guard me against credulity and the illusion of knowledge, and assist me to bridge the chasm between laboratory bench and hospital ward. They would prevent me from becoming a note-taking field worker who contented himself with the mere reporting of detailed but uninterpretable examples. I could help them embed their discoveries in stories. Medical science was richly various and very messy but its spirit was divine. To be successful it required openness, freedom to disagree without censure, and a healthy disrespect for authority.

7

– Contraband –

I n 1977, a polythene bag full of white powder was smuggled through Heathrow airport by Professor Merton Sandler in his deep-pocketed 'flasher's mac'. It was a cargo of scientific contraband that was to give me a critical edge on New York competitors and launch me on a journey of sacrificial investigation. L-deprenil (E-250), an inhibitor of monoamine oxidase, was a gift from Josef Knoll, Head of Pharmacology at the Semmelweis University in Budapest. He was convinced that his molecule had enormous clinical potential as a psychic energiser and nerve tonic.

The monoamine oxidases are a family of enzymes responsible for the physiological breakdown of a number of chemical messengers including serotonin, noradrenaline and dopamine, believed to be important in the regulation of mood. They had first become a target for psychopharmacological investigation in the 1950s after a group of patients dying from tuberculosis had been given a new drug called iproniazid (Marsilid). A newspaper reported how some of these consumptives had started to 'dance for joy' in the corridors of Sea View Sanatorium on Staten Island. This surprising occurrence led on to a few curious psychiatrists conducting trials with iproniazid on small groups of patients with psychotic depression. Some of the desperate volunteers, who had been resistant to all other therapeutic approaches, reported an increased sense of wellbeing and vitality.

Iproniazid was soon being trumpeted in the press as the first specific 'antidepressant' and between April 1957 and February 1958 an estimated 380,000 psychiatric patients were treated with the drug in the United States. Not long after its introduction, a neurologist reported that every time his wife took iproniazid and then ate cheese, she developed severe headaches and her blood pressure went up to dangerously high levels. This complication of treatment became known as 'the cheese effect' and after a few patients had tragically died from haemorrhages into their brain, the regulatory authorities imposed a dietary embargo of tyramine (found in strong cheeses and some other foodstuffs) as a prerequisite for the continuing use of the drug.

After the discovery of severe dopamine loss in Parkinson's disease in 1960 the combination of iproniazid with L-DOPA seemed a logical pharmacological strategy for relief of the shaking palsy. By delaying its enzymatic breakdown and reducing the rapid turnover of the remaining 'natural' dopamine in the brain, monoamine oxidase inhibitors might be expected to enhance chemical transmission. Unfortunately, severe elevations of blood pressure occurred similar to those seen with tyramine-containing foods and precluded the routine use of what otherwise might have been a useful therapeutic marriage.

The existence of two distinct forms of monoamine oxidase known as Type A and Type B was suspected by the time Joseph Knoll's 'present' arrived in London and I hoped that L-deprenil ('depression nil') and its anagram 'end peril' might prove to be an omen.

Merton Sandler had assured me that deprenil was 'safe as houses' and I willingly agreed to become part of my own experiment. I took 10 milligrams a day for a week at the end of which time I was 'admitted' to a side cubicle on Ward 5.2 where a colleague plied me with escalating doses of tyramine. Tyramine is a substance that is found in minute quantities in the brain, and in large amounts can displace stored monoamines leading to elevations in blood pressure. The purpose of my self-experimentation was to determine whether deprenil, in contrast to the first wave of non-selective monoamine oxidase inhibitors, could be taken safely with tyramine-rich foodstuffs like Gorgonzola cheese, pickled herrings, chocolate, Chianti wine, pulses and Marmite.

This 'single subject research' conducted in the garret of the Cruciform Building on Gower Street allowed me to experience what it must be like for a patient to volunteer for a trial with an untested drug. L-deprenil made me more alert, created pleasant waking dreams and induced a disarming fatuous euphoria. I was full of beans and my wife felt I ought to continue on the drug permanently. Measurement of my monoamine oxidase levels in blood platelets confirmed that deprenil had long lasting and powerful selective inhibitory effects on the Type B species of monoamine oxidase. I had also been able to tolerate 'industrial' doses of tyramine without any increase in my blood pressure or headaches.

It was also important to determine if L-deprenil could be used safely with L-DOPA before clinical trials could be contemplated. To my relief, administration of 10mg of deprenil to six L-DOPA treated volunteers with Parkinson's disease did not cause hypertension. The endgame was in view.

Understandably, the United Kingdom Medicines Commission felt unable to formally sanction a trial with an illegally acquired substance but common sense prevailed and tacit approval to proceed was granted on the proviso that we obtained ethical approval from the hospital and informed consent from the patients. My main scientific partner on the project, John Elsworth, then got one of his pharmacist friends to produce a few thousand capsules, each containing 5 mg deprenil from Sandler's bag of white powder without charge. There was no shortage of volunteers desperate to try deprenil even though we had virtually no safety data other than our own experience with the drug. Despite the miracle of L-DOPA, Parkinson's disease was still a crippling handicap and a great deal was at stake.

The trial went smoothly and I was able to confirm that deprenil could be used safely in combination with

L-DOPA and without the need for tyramine dietary restriction. I also showed with the help of diaries filled in by the patients that the drug could increase the duration of benefit obtained from each dose of L-DOPA. A small number of the volunteers were in the very earliest stages of the disease and had not yet been given L-DOPA. On 10mg a day some felt much more vigilant, optimistic and energetic and described improvement in their speed of movement.

I concluded that l-deprenil was easy to use and could help to iron out the end of dose deterioration ('wearing offs') seen in some patients on chronic L-DOPA treatment, but it was much less potent than bromocriptine and certainly not the wondrous cure that I had hoped for.

Following the publication of our results in *The Lancet,* the most prestigious general medicine journal in Britain, I was encouraged to present the data at International Symposia on Parkinson's disease and it was at one of these – a meeting in Vienna – that I was first introduced to Doctor Josef Knoll. He was a tanned, extremely fit-looking, fifty-five-year-old who spoke English fluently with a thick Hungarian accent. When he spoke his voice was charged with emotion and long passages of words were uttered without break, with the *v* sound sometimes replacing the letter *w*. He told me that he had been taking deprenil for several years and that the drug had greatly improved both his mental sharpness and sexual vitality. He was in no doubt that deprenil could lengthen lifespan. What impressed me most on that first meeting was his dynamism and certainty. He came over as God-like and infallible.

I later learned from Gerald Stern that Knoll had survived Auschwitz where he had seen his parents die, Buchenwald, and finally ridden out the notorious Dachau death train before being liberated by the Americans, weighing just 39 kg. After World War II, he had tried to make sense of his experience in the Nazi concentration camps by studying innate and acquired drives in laboratory animals. As part of this work he had trained rats to search for and jump to the rim of a 30 cm high glass cylinder and then crawl inside. This acquired drive had become so powerful that it could override the rats' instinctive appetites. In several related experiments he used amphetamines as a way to ignite the brain's engine. 'Speed' excited the midbrain to release noradrenaline and dopamine, two chemical messengers that he believed were critical for the process of transforming novel experiences into acquired drives and ingrained habits.

Within eighteen months of our *Lancet* paper being published, investigators in New York and Finland reported similar clinical results. Whether an experiment is carried out on one blinkered scientist or a thousand volunteers, it still requires validation from an external source and it was a great relief to receive confirmation of my results.

Deprenil soon became a popular adjuvant treatment for Parkinson's disease. The recommended dose was 5–10 mg a day although it had seemed from the clinical pharmacological studies I had undertaken that 10 mg once a month might be more than adequate to prevent the metabolic degradation of dopamine in the brain. Despite its popularity with doctors and patients, no large pharmaceutical company showed any interest in buying and marketing it.

The arrival of bromocriptine and deprenil into clinical practice in the late seventies provided an embarrassment of riches in comparison to therapeutic options for other common neurological diseases like Alzheimer's and multiple sclerosis, but led to increasing uncertainty among neurologists about the best way to initiate treatment in Parkinson's disease. In an attempt to try to answer this dilemma, the Parkinson's Disease Research Group of the United Kingdom was set up as a registered charity in 1982. Its remit was to enlist a group of neurologists and some specialists in the care of the elderly to participate in a trial in which hundreds of untreated patients would be recruited and randomised to one of three initial treatments – L-DOPA, deprenil combined with L-DOPA, or bromocriptine. The patients would be followed at three-monthly intervals throughout the entire course of their illness.

Academic curiosity and a hankering to resolve

uncertainties in clinical practice were the motivations for the eighty hospital specialists who recruited patients from their National Health Service practices. Investigators paid their own travel expenses to attend the meetings and gave up considerable amounts of their own time to take part. Most clinical trials sponsored by the pharmaceutical industry focused only on short-term efficacy and excluded patients over the age of seventy-five and also those with co-existing medical conditions like cancer and stroke. In sharp contrast, the primary interest of this trial centred on whether one of the treatments was superior in extending life expectancy. Although a placebo arm was not included in its design, we felt that the long follow-up and liberal inclusion criteria would ultimately prove to be great strengths of the study.

Not long after the UK Parkinson's Research Group had started to recruit patients, six heroin addicts presented to emergency rooms around the Bay Area of San Francisco with signs of acute parkinsonism. Neurological detective work revealed that all of them had recently injected the same batch of a designer opioid called MPPP. It was determined that the 'kitchen chemist' had taken a shortcut in the drug's synthesis and the sloppy batch he had sold to his clients was contaminated with a non-narcotic called MPTP.

MPTP had first been synthesised in 1947 as a

potential analgesic by the Hofmann La Roche Company in Switzerland. Immobility and tremor had occurred during testing in laboratory monkeys and two of six human volunteers who were given MPTP mysteriously died. Two scientists working with other companies also came down with 'MPTP sickness' and research into the compound was abandoned.

The tragedy of the Santa Clara frozen addicts led to a frenzy of interest in MPTP but this time as a toxin rather than as a potential painkiller. Scientists showed that an active metabolite of MPTP, a slightly altered compound called MPP+, could destroy the melanin containing nerve cells in the midbrain and induce a behavioural syndrome in monkeys that closely resembled Parkinson's disease. At the very least it was hoped that the MPTP paradigm would serve as an improved animal model for testing possible new treatments.

Then an experiment was carried out that would rock the Parkinson's disease community. Jan Chiba, a graduate student working in San Francisco, was curious to find out how the protoxin MPTP was converted in the brain to MPP+. He hypothesised that MPTP entered the brain where it was mistaken by monoamine oxidase for dopamine and metabolised by the enzyme to MPP+.

In a series of test tube experiments, Chiba was able to confirm his notion and show that two monoamine oxidase inhibitors, pargyline and deprenil, completely prevented the conversion of MPTP to the toxic species

MPP+. William Langston, who had been one of the doctors to first examine the frozen addicts, then initiated further experiments in which monkeys were pretreated with deprenil and showed that it completely protected their dopamine pathways from the toxin MPP+. It was proposed that deprenil might prevent the accumulation of toxic free radicals like hydrogen peroxide in dopamine nerve cells, and exposure to pesticides with chemical structures similar to MPTP became a serious contender for the cause of Parkinson's disease.

Largely as a result of these compelling findings, the National Institutes of Health in Bethesda, USA, agreed to fund the largest trial ever carried out in Parkinson's disease on eight hundred previously untreated patients with the primary aims of determining if either deprenil or Vitamin E could retard disease deterioration (The Parkinson Study Group DATATOP trial).

The results of this trial were published in 1989 in the *New England Journal of Medicine* accompanied by a glowing editorial indicating that deprenil in a dose of 10 milligrams per day could delay the onset of disability associated with early untreated Parkinson's disease and might prove to be the first ever scientifically proven neuroprotective agent. The news release heralded:

Miami Beach, May 2nd, 1990 – A new drug therapy used in the early stages of Parkinson's disease delays the need for L-DOPA therapy and should enable patients to enjoy longer periods of productive employment, family life and well being.

Doctor Langston, one of the trial investigators, told the press, 'For the first time, there is hope for patients with Parkinson's disease.'

In the November 1989 edition of the *Philadelphia Enquirer* another participant, Dr Hurtig, said, 'Doctors should consider giving the drug to all Parkinson's disease patients.'

8

– Crushed Hopes –

As a result of the preliminary findings of the DATATOP study, it became widely accepted that deprenil might be able to stop Parkinson's disease spreading through the brain. Knoll's self-experimentation had received scientific validation from a highly reputable group of investigators.

Then, in 1993, further long-term analyses of the trial cast doubt on this understandable outburst of misplaced optimism. The new data clearly demonstrated that the disability scores had diminished in some of the deprenil treated patients. This raised an alternative possibility as to why the patients on deprenil had been able to delay starting L-DOPA. A modification of the original conclusions was necessary, with a more guarded interpretation of the findings. It seemed to me that the Parkinson Study Group's careful and rigorous observations had finally undermined their own unbridled enthusiasm.

In our 1977 *Lancet* paper we had drawn attention to improvement seen in some previously untreated patients with deprenil. If the North American DATATOP investigators had paid more attention to this report they may have at least considered an alternative trial design. My thoughts turned back to the numerous instances where respected American colleagues had refused to reference important science published outside their own back yard. If the findings hadn't appeared in a journal published in the United States of America then they weren't worth reading!

When William Landau, a distinguished neurological elder, had the temerity to challenge the validity of the DATATOP conclusions, he was pilloried in the correspondence section of *Neurology*:

Certainly, Landau is entitled to express his opinion, but he should not be exempt from peer review or contemporaneous response. Landau offered not a whit of novel, substantive criticism. Rather, he played to the crowd with innuendo, cute turns of phrase and, unfortunately, a large measure of either intentional obfuscation or lack of clear understanding. Landau's article served only one useful function: it illustrates the need for proper editorial review.

I largely agreed with Landau's criticisms and envied 'his cute turns of phrase'. Almost all the leading figures in American Parkinson's disease research had taken part in the DATATOP study so it was left to a senior statesman of neurology to provide a salutary word of caution about the increasing unacceptable use of spin in medical research

The United Kingdom Parkinson's Disease Research Group reported its preliminary six-year findings in the

British Medical Journal in 1995. Contrary to expectations, the group of patients who had received deprenil combined with L-DOPA had an increased mortality rate. This cast serious doubt on deprenil's neuro-restorative potential.

By this time, I had been elected the convenor and Honorary Secretary for the Group and as spokesman for the trial found myself in the invidious position of being the first person to put a dint in the charmed reputation of a drug that had given so many patients hope.

Neurologists and patients wanted to believe, and had clung to the notion that deprenil might slow the march of Parkinson's disease even after the DATATOP volte-face. Deprenil was too alluring to abandon easily and had become a petrified truth. It was now also being promulgated as a possible treatment for Alzheimer's disease, depression and fatigue. Professional boxers and body builders were taking it illicitly to enhance performance, and in Canada it had been added to dog food to promote canine vitality.

In contrast to the DATATOP trial that had been widely defended as impeccable peer-reviewed scientific research conducted by a group of experienced and sophisticated clinical trialists, a torrent of criticism engulfed our findings. Particularly vituperative letters were received by the journal from medical statisticians and some members of the United States Parkinson's Study Group who argued that our methodology and statistical analysis were both inherently flawed. In their view, the lack of a placebo arm for at least the first six months of the trial was a serious shortcoming. Doubt was also cast on the competence of specialists in geriatric medicine to adequately assess disability in Parkinson's disease.

Under threat of subpoena I was summoned to give telephone evidence to the United States Food and Drug Administration (FDA). A barrage of hostile questions from regulators and lawyers rained down. The FDA also requested permission and had legal authority to investigate all the paperwork relating to the trial. I felt relieved that our main end point depended on death certification rather than the unreliable clinical rating scales that are even today the only practical way to measure change in physical handicap in Parkinson's disease. The French Government, on the other hand, wanted to ban deprenil rather than protect it and I was asked to provide a confidential report on the methods and results of our trial. I felt vulnerable and exposed and received no support from the General Medical Council, the Medical Defence Union or the University.

The Parkinson's Disease Research Group of the United Kingdom acted promptly and set up an independent data monitoring panel to look for an explanation for the cause of the increased and unexpected mortality seen on the L-DOPA/deprenil combination.

The commonest cause of death in patients with Parkinson's disease, as judged from death certification, is pneumonia, either from bacterial or viral infection or aspiration of food into the lungs, but there was extremely limited historical data available to inform the committee. A careful scrutiny of all the death certificates and the autopsy data from those few patients who had received post-mortems, failed to reveal a single explanation for the increased loss of life seen with the L-DOPA/ deprenil combination treatment. In our paper we speculated that the increased number of deaths might have occurred in a subgroup of elderly patients who were at risk of heart rhythm disturbances or drops in blood pressure as a consequence of cardiovascular co-morbidity that would have excluded them from drug company sponsored trials.

The findings continued to generate debate and acrimony for years. Opponents tried to expunge our *British Medical Journal* paper from memory by performing half-baked meta-analyses and systematic reviews. Despite Orion Pharma's attempts to limit the financial damage of the UK Parkinson's Disease Research Group trial, our results had dented the deprenil business and the drug's sales fell markedly and rapidly in the United Kingdom.

Josef Knoll never forgave me and in his book *How Deprenyl Slows Brain Aging*, published in his 87th year in 2012, he wrote:

An example of a multicentre clinical trial in which the improper combination of levodopa with deprenil led to confusion and misinterpretation is the one performed by the United Kingdom Parkinson's Disease Group of the United Kingdom (UK-PDRG) (Lees 1995). Quite unexpectedly this group published an alarming paper claiming that parkinsonian patients treated with L-DOPA combined with deprenil show an increased mortality in comparison with the patients treated with L-DOPA alone. The finding was in striking contradiction to all other studies published in a variety of countries.

I wished that I had had the opportunity to emphasise to him our very cautious interpretation of the interim results and the Group's determination to continue the trial after re-randomising the deprenil patients to one of the other two arms. Several years later we were able to show that there was no lasting advantage to starting treatment with either deprenil or bromocriptine and that L-DOPA, contrary to popular opinion, was not toxic, a view that is now generally accepted by all national guidelines and evidence based reviews. Our trial had been conducted on a shoestring budget using the research resource of the National Health Service and neither the investigators nor patients received any form of remuneration. It was also one of the very first trials to emphasise the absolute necessity of increasing the length of follow up in Parkinson's disease trials to a minimum of ten years.

Up until his death, Knoll continued to believe

and deny. He was a high priest in possession of a great power. I became his academic enemy because our data had contradicted his starry-eyed view of deprenil. The most charitable explanation I could find for his behaviour was that he was protecting his commercial interest and that he had fallen out of love with the scientific process. His YouTube video, which provided an overview of his book, resembled a sales pitch. The idea of a midbrain enhancer delaying brain aging seemed even more way out now than it had done at the time when I still wanted to believe. I could now see all too clearly the detrimental effect of hype in medicine. The scientific hard sell inevitably underwrote an insecure investment.

9

– Rainforest Science –

I n the sixth form at school, I had been introduced to the work of Richard Spruce, a self-taught moss and liverwort collector. *Notes of a Botanist on the Amazon and Andes*, compiled by Alfred Russel Wallace from Spruce's personal notebooks, letters and diaries, became my guiding light. Spruce had criss-crossed vast stretches of the Amazon jungle at the same time as Wallace and the entomologist Henry Bates and despite their fierce competitiveness and need to collect specimens to earn a living, these professional naturalists, all from humble backgrounds, had remained friends long after they had returned to England. All three had been forced to descend into a primal chaos to search for a liberating, rational truth.

Spruce was a negligible interloper on a peculiar errand, but there were times when the portentousness of the Amazon basin had made him feel like a fallen comet, lost and scattered over the earth's crust. In the upper Uaupés almost every plant he collected was an unrecorded species. He wrote to George Bentham at Kew:

I well recollect how the banks of the river had become clad with flowers, as it were by some sudden magic, and how I said to myself as I scanned the lofty trees with wistful and disappointed eyes, 'there goes a new Dipteryx – there goes a new Qualea – there goes a new the Lord knows what!' until I could no longer bear the sight and covering up my face with my hands, I resigned myself to the sorrowful reflection that I must leave all these fine things to waste their sweetness on the jungle air.

– *Notes of a Botanist on the Amazon and Andes*

Some days he would spend hours rooted to a single spot admiring the arrangements of lichens. What seemed to the uncultured eye like a mind-numbing wilderness had provided him with an opportunity to write his name into history. On some evenings he carried out self-experimentation in an attempt to verify the medicinal and magical properties claimed by the Indians for the plants he had pressed.

Spruce risked his life in order to discover and study new species of flora. Every lichen, with its millions of emerald ears and golden mouths, held secrets that challenged his erudition. The interrelationships of plants informed him about the world in which he lived. Spruce's life goal was to expose the laws of nature. He considered plants to be sentient beings that beautified the earth. In a letter to his friend, Daniel Hanbury, he wrote:

It is true that the Hepaticae have hardly as yet yielded any substance to man capable of stupefying him, or of forcing his stomach to empty its contents, nor are they good for food; but if man cannot torture them to his uses or abuse, they are infinitely useful where God has placed them [. . .] and they are, at the least, useful to, and beautiful in, themselves – surely the primary motive for every individual existence.

In this green Mars he saw things that he knew had never been seen before by the trained eye – sensational plant forms that he feared he would never behold again. His descriptions left me with an indelible impression of the convulsive beauty of the forest. There was an integrity and essential goodness about his life and a refreshing innocence. His work epitomised the romance and openness of science and brought biology alive.

Spruce alerted me to how much of the unknown the darkness still held but this should not deter me in my attempts to observe more clearly. He taught me that science was precious and must be pure, that fieldwork had an important part to play in discovery and that unshakeable faith and tenacity were needed to make headway. Despite his abhorrence of any attempt to reduce the Amazon to a list of potential commodities he also hinted in his logbooks that the plants of the rainforest held most of the secrets to understanding and manipulating the chemical systems of the human brain.

Long after I had given up all hopes of following Spruce into the rainforest, I ran into him for a second time in the course of researching the history of monoamine oxidase inhibitors for the introductory chapters of my doctoral thesis on deprenil. Nine years after his reluctant return from South America, Spruce wrote an article entitled 'On Some Remarkable Narcotics of the Amazon Valley and Orinoco' published in *Ocean Highways, The Geographical Magazine* in 1873. In the article, he related how in November 1852, while staying in the village of Panuré, situated at the base of two treacherous narrow channels on the Rio Uaupés, he had befriended some Tukano Indians and after he had gained their confidence through his fluency in their language, he was invited to attend their Feast of Gifts. He arrived at dusk in a place called Urubú-coará (The Vulture's Nest) four miles above the rapids to be greeted by the doleful sound of trumpets. In the intermissions between the tribesmen's communal dancing, an Indian carrying two calabashes of caapi would run from the thatched house murmuring 'Mo-mo-mo-mo-mo-mo', then squat to allow the Tukanos gathered in a semi-circle to imbibe the greenish yellow liquid. Within a few minutes of drinking the potion, Spruce recorded that the tribesmen turned pale, retched and began to shiver. Some broke into a sweat and bellowed out in anger, beating their weapons threateningly on the ground while shouting out the names of their enemies. Calmness then descended and some of the intoxicated men closed their glazed eyes briefly before the dancing resumed. Spruce noted that the women were not allowed to witness the feast and were forced to hide away inside the long ancestral house. He also observed that although five or six caapi rituals occurred throughout the night, it was extremely uncommon for any one Indian to drink the brew on more than one occasion.

Spruce was offered a half measure of the bitter concoction, followed by liberal quantities of manioc beer and palm wine. He was also instructed to smoke a two-foot long tobacco cigar. The overall effect of this heady cocktail of alkaloids was sedation and a nauseous inebriation, forcing him to retire to his hammock.

He made it his business to learn that the most important ingredient of caapi was a fast growing liana with a thick, double helical stem and an alternate pinnate leaf arrangement. The vine had an attractive inflorescence of tiny pinkish white flowers with five sepals and five petals. After the Tukanos had collected the climbing plant from the forest, the lower part of its stem was beaten in a mortar with some water and then concentrated by boiling. The mixture was then sieved to remove any fibre and stored in a sacred urn.

Spruce collected some fresh specimens of the twiner that he had found growing in a manioc plot and dispatched them to the Royal Botanical Gardens at Kew for classification and analysis in March 1853. On their eventual arrival at Kew, George Bentham, the systematic botanist, was able to confirm Spruce's opinion that these voucher samples were a hitherto unclassified species of Malpighiaceae and endorse his proposed provisional Latin name of *Banisteria caapi*.

The following year Spruce again watched the ceremonial use of caapi, this time among the Guahibo Indians of the Upper Orinoco, and noted that they

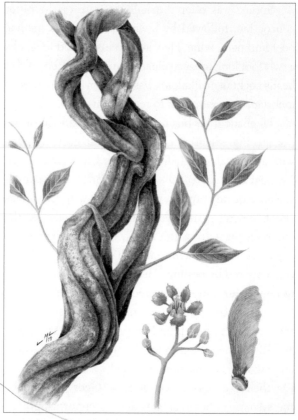

Banisteriopsis caapi, the source of yagé

also chewed the dry stem. He was now convinced that the caapi brew contained a rapidly acting potent substance with divinatory properties quite distinct from opium, Indian hemp and coca and he expressed hope that the samples he had dispatched to Kew would be analysed.

A few years after *Notes of a Botanist* had finally been published in 1908 and twenty years after Spruce's death, the first chemical secrets of caapi were revealed to the world. *Banisteria* samples were sent by chemists at the University of Bogotá to E. Merck, a pharmaceutical company based in Germany, who had developed a major research interest in the medicinal potential of mind-bending molecules. The scientists working at Merck sent some of the material to a freelance Berlin pharmacologist called Louis Lewin, who isolated a new alkaloid he called banisterine from the stems. A few years later the Merck chemists showed that banisterine and two other pharmacologically active extracts from the vine, tentatively labelled yageine and telepathine, were all chemically indistinguishable from a nitrogenous molecule called harmine.

One evening in 1952, while waiting for a train at Grand Central Station in Manhattan, William Burroughs read about yagé (also known as caapi and ayahuasca) in a magazine. The article described how the 'vine of the soul' allowed the Indian shaman to foresee the future and communicate with the minds of his ancestors. It went on to describe how a medicine man from the Kofán tribe had been able to envision the city of Copenhagen including some of its street signs and describe them to a Danish explorer. After renouncing psychoanalysis, Burroughs had become increasingly interested in extrasensory perception and clairvoyance and was intrigued by the plant's alleged pharmacological effects.

He then carried out research into the plant in the New York Public Library. There he learned that *Banisteriopsis caapi* was a fast growing liana with a thick stem that could reach a length of sixty feet and that the inner bark was the main source of the hallucinating narcotic. He was disappointed by the dearth of first-hand accounts of yagé's psychotropic effects and wrote to his former hypnotherapist Dr Wolberg in the hope of obtaining further information. In the letter Burroughs wrote, 'I don't know your opinion but I consider telepathy an established fact'. Wolberg informed Burroughs that yagé was under wraps because the US Army were conducting secret experiments with the plant.

Unphased by the relative lack of data, Burroughs embarked on his first serious attempt 'to dig yagé' in 1953. Not long after his arrival in Bogotá, he had the good fortune to bump into Doctor Richard Schultes (in *The Yage Letters* he is disguised as 'Doctor Schindler'). Schultes was an American ethnobotanist who had graduated from Harvard a year after Burroughs and had then spent most of the next twelve years sailing down the tributaries of the North Western Amazon in a portable aluminium craft. Schultes' close collaboration with plant chemists in Boston had helped to reveal the medicinal secrets of at least two hundred indigenous plants and his exacting fieldwork had culminated in important new insights into 'the second sight' of the Amazon Indian. At their first meeting at the Universidad Nacional de Colombia, Schultes had pulled out a dry, wrinkled piece of caapi stem and told Burroughs that under the plant's influence he had experienced blue and grey colours.

Schultes' Victorian decorum, his habit of voting for the Queen of England in the American Presidential elections and his dogged insistence on the use of systematic botanical names had made some of his Harvard students question whether he might be the living embodiment of the Yorkshire-born Richard Spruce.

Burroughs then left Bogotá alone on an eventful five-week journey to Puerto Asis in the Putumayo region of Colombia. As well as having his first experience with yagé he was mugged, thrown in a police cell, contracted malaria and witnessed first-hand the civil war that had been raging in the countryside between the Conservatives and the Liberals (La Violencia) for more than five years. On 28 February 1953, he wrote to his ally, the poet Allen Ginsberg, from the Hotel Niza in the Andean mountainside town of Pasto, describing his first half-baked experience of yagé:

That night I had a vivid dream in color of the green jungle and a red sunset [. . .] Also a composite city familiar to me but I could not quite place it. Part New York, part Mexico City and part Lima which I had not seen at this time.

–*The Yage Letters*

After his return to Bogotá, Schultes provided Burroughs with the opportunity to attach himself with the Anglo-Cocoa Commission that was about to begin a thousand mile round trip expedition into the rainforests of Southern Colombia. On this trek Burroughs was to learn a great deal more about yagé. Schultes told him that his father, a plumber, had read him excerpts of *Notes of a Botanist on the Amazon and the Andes* when he was ill as a teenager and it was this that had led him into the jungle. He told Burroughs that the Indians saw the caapi stem as a cord that connected them with their mythical past. In order to communicate with the invisible world of the Milky Way and their ancestors, they needed to pass from one cosmic plane to another. He also told him that when a Desãna Indian feels ill he asks who he has annoyed, not what he might have eaten.

In the municipality of Mocoa, Burroughs was introduced to an elderly baby-faced Ingano medicine man who invited him to partake in a yagé ceremony. The shaman lived in a thatched shack inside which was a shrine with a picture of the Virgin Mary, a cross, feathers, a wooden effigy and a few small packages tied with ribbons. The Indian took a swig from Burroughs' bottle of aguardiente and then sat down on the dirt floor behind a bowl set on a tripod. He started to chant the words 'Yagé Pintar' and then got up and swished a light broom on Burroughs' shoulders to whisk away the evil spirits. The Indian then took a drink from the bowl and poured some of the dark oily liquid into a dirty red plastic cup. Burroughs drunk the bitter concoction and within two minutes felt vertiginous, nauseous and inebriated. He then saw some blue flashes, the hut took on a far-Pacific look with Easter Island heads, and as he stumbled about in an uncoordinated fashion he saw squawking larval forms surrounded by an azure haze. A few hours after he had taken the drink, in fear of an impending convulsion he was forced to take the barbiturate Nembutal as an antidote. By first light he was well enough to walk back down the mountainside to the Hotel America but was still experiencing showers of blue flashes. He told members of the expedition that he considered the shaman to be a deceitful charlatan who specialised in bumping off gringos.

Burroughs learned from Schultes that the Inganos and Cofans crushed the vine with a rock and often mixed it with leaves from other plants, whereas close to the Brazilian border on the upper Uaupés, the Tukanos that Spruce had befriended scraped shavings from the vine and allowed it to mull alone for several hours in cold water. One of Schultes' Indian guides from the Rio Uaupés prepared this pure version for Burroughs, who sipped it over an hour but the effect was disappointing, with only a few blue-grey flashes and mild erotism that he likened to the effects of marijuana.

On his return to the Colombian capital, Burroughs continued his scientific investigations in the run-down laboratory at the Botanical Institute of the university, with the intention of distilling the active substance from the nauseating oils and resins. Schultes provided him with a published extraction method but the brown feathery residue Burroughs managed to isolate from the crate of dried yagé he had brought back with him proved to be disappointingly devoid of hallucinatory effect. He wrote again to Allen Ginsberg saying that only the fresh vine had the real kick and that yageine or harmine extracts were a pale replica, devoid of a vital volatile element.

He then headed for Peru in search of more yagé experiences and in Pucallpa, on the banks of the Rio Ucayali, he learned that a team of Russian scientists had visited the region in 1927 and shipped a ton of yagé back to Moscow. Burroughs was now certain there was an undercover story to write relating to brainwashing experiments with the devil's vine that implicated both the KGB and the CIA.

His experiences with yagé in Peru were far more intense than anything he had experienced in Colombia. He described scintillating diamonds that turned like dancers on the tips of remote freeways, slow undulating celestial waves ('blue spirit'), multitudes, and monochromatic clouds racing across the night sky. He later wrote that the kick was seeing things from a special angle: it was purely visceral and permitted a temporary freedom from the claims of the ageing, terrified, cautious flesh. Writing hurriedly in pencil from the Hotel Pucallpa on 18 June 1953, Burroughs orders Ginsberg to hold back the scientific Yagé article he had sent him (in which he had stated that only the fresh liana was responsible for the hallucinogenic effects):

Hold the presses! . . . I am now prepared to believe the Brujos do have secrets, and that Yage alone is quite different from Yage prepared with the leaves and plants the Brujos add to it.

In a letter to Allen Ginsberg posted from Lima on July 8 1953, he spoke of yagé being a 'blue drug' and a 'night drug':

Like I say it is like nothing else. This is not the chemical lift of C, the sexless horribly sane stasis of junk, the vegetable nightmare of peyote, or the humorous silliness of weed. This is an instant overwhelming rape of the senses.
– *Letters 1945–1959*

Burroughs had defined junk in *Naked Lunch* as a generic term for opium and its morphine derivatives, including all its synthetic forms such as heroin, Demerol, Palfium, Eukodal and Paregoric. Yagé was different and the most powerful drug he had ever taken.

On July 10 he wrote once more to Ginsberg from Lima:

Yage is space-time travel. The room seems to shake and vibrate with motion . . . You make migrations, incredible journeys through deserts and jungles and mountains.

– *The Yage Letters*

In Pucallpa, Burroughs had got to know the local 'doctor,' a young man named Saboya ('a doctor works cures whereas a 'brujo' deals in both cures and curses'), who poured some yagé out of a beer bottle into a cup and whistled over it. After Burroughs had drunk from the cup, a blue substance invaded his body, his jaw clamped tight and he developed convulsive tremors of the limbs. Saboya told Burroughs 'I have no enemies, I turn them all into friends'. Burroughs learned that the vine of the soul helped to correct any disharmony the Indian felt with the forest. In their universal womb the visible and invisible become of equal authenticity and when they return to conscious unreality they incorporate the shapes and patterns of their visions into their forest world. After several more ceremonies, Saboya eventually agreed to divulge to Burroughs the trade secrets of his yagé preparation:

He mashes pieces of the fresh cut vine and boils two hours with the leaves of another plant tentatively identified by a Peruvian botanist as Palicourea Species Rubiaceae. The effect of Yage, prepared in this manner is qualitatively different from cold-water infusion of Yage alone, or Yage cooked alone. The other leaf is essential to realize the full effect of the drug. Whether it is itself active, or merely serves as a catalysing agent, I do not know. This matter needs the attention of a chemist.

– *The Yage Letters*

Burroughs bought several bottles of the magic brew from the medicine man and observed that after repetitive yagé use, tolerance to the debilitating nausea developed which persisted for several months after abstinence. Burroughs now associated the cerebral nausea with motion sickness and inner space travel. Through the power of yagé he had glimpsed a supernatural state of being that provided him with a gateway into a proximate closed-off past. Daily living was an illusion or a dream, and if he were to free himself from the dementia of Middle America he would need to stop questioning and give up all attempts to explain. He must now eschew the results business and stop trying to seek answers in terms of cause and effect and prediction. The mechanical acquisition of facts was a waste of time, at least where the Amazon was concerned. Yagé had permanently altered his metabolism and in so doing altered the constant scanning pattern of his former reality. It would provide him with a ladder to the Magical Universe. He later wrote that his exposure to the liana had been more effective in straightening him out than a hundred hours of psychoanalysis.

Burroughs remained in contact with Doctor Schultes and posted him a Christmas card and a voucher specimen of the plant that enhanced the effects of *Banisteriopsis.* In January 1955, he wrote to Ginsberg from Tangier about his disappointment that Schultes, whom he greatly respected, had stopped corresponding with him.

In 'Letter from a Master Addict to Dangerous Drugs', published in the *British Journal of Addiction* in 1956, Burroughs wrote:

About five pieces of vine each eight inches long are needed for one person. The vine is crushed and boiled for two or more hours with the leaves of a bush identified as Palicourea sp. Rubiacea.

Twelve years after Schultes had severed contact with Burroughs, The United States Department of Health, Education and Welfare organized a symposium entitled 'Ethnopharmacologic Search for Psychoactive Drugs' in San Francisco. At this meeting Schultes informed the scientific world that the strongest yagé fireworks occurred when the bark of *Banisteriopsis caapi* was mixed with the leaves of the perennial shrub *Psychotria viridis*, known by the Indians as *chacrona,* or with another plant they called *chacropanga*. The Proceedings of this conference became a classic in psychedelic literature, although Schultes' seminal paper was largely ignored in the frenzy of interest in LSD-25 and psilocybin.

The chemical secrets of yagé had also now been partly unlocked. Sidney Udenfriend, a Brooklyn born biochemist working at the National Institutes of Health in Bethesda, Maryland, had shown that harmine, the alkaloid believed to be responsible for yagé's pharmacological effects, was a reversible monoamine oxidase inhibitor which could impede the physiological destruction of serotonin in the brain. The leaves of *chacrona* and *chacropanga* both contained the short acting psychoactive serotonin compound N, N-dimethyltryptamine (DMT). The combination of these two molecules could create a prismatic firework display in the mind's eye.

A year after the San Francisco conference, Schultes visited the Royal Botanical Gardens at Kew and analysed Spruce's samples of caapi. In the learned journal *De plantis toxicariis e mundo novo tropicale commentationes* he reported that even after more than a century of preservation the stems of B.caapi still contained a substantial quantity of harmine. In the same article he acknowledged William Burroughs' one and only contribution to ethnobotany:

The utilisation of Psychotria viridis was first reported in 1967, but an earlier herbarium collection had indicated its use as an additive with b.caapi (William Burroughs s.n.).

What continued to nag away at Schultes was how Indians in many different regions of the Amazon had learned to successfully pair these particular plants for their sacred practices. Could the instinct of the jaguar or elemental plant forces have led the ancient civilizations to a synergy that then gradually spread through the forest? Could the living communion of the Amazon have created plant-human symbioses that went far beyond natural selection or was it all simply a result of trial and error?

I felt justified in concluding the historical review in my doctoral thesis by crowning Richard Spruce the father of monoamine oxidase inhibition. He had identified B. caapi as the single most important ingredient of caapi but had also hinted that other plants could be added to the potion. Richard Schultes was the first to scientifically detail the medicine man's trade secrets but William Burroughs also deserved an honourable mention. In Burroughs' world no scientific law was perfect or certain. *Naked Lunch* and *The Yage Letters* had tuned me into an unsentimental form of rain forest science.

My intense period of scientific research was now over and I resumed my clinical training at the National Hospital, Queen Square – the cradle of British neurology where I had been so inspired on my return from Paris by teachers like MacDonald Critchley. Ascetic yet charismatic, tall and always impeccably dressed, Critchley cast an imposing and elegant figure on his visits to the bedside of the neurologically sick. By the time I 'got on the house' he was in his eighties and retired from the National Health Service but he was still a sought-after second opinion and my new chiefs would sometimes ask me to go and discuss difficult cases with him. After several visits to his small third floor apartment next to the hospital, I plucked up courage to ask him about his early interest in visual hallucinations. With his arresting turn of phrase and polished prose he told me that after reading Louis Lewin's book *Phantastica: A Classic Survey on the Use and Abuse of Mind-Altering Plants*, he had taken 0.2 mg of mescaline sulphate under experimental circumstances. He then drew my attention to his 1931 article on the subject entitled 'Some Forms of Drug Addiction: Mescalism'. Towards the end of the essay, Critchley had speculated about mescaline's potential as a therapy:

Lastly, the scope of mescal in the field of therapeutics is almost unexplored. The Indian uses this plant for every manner of ailment; and indeed attempts have been made to introduce peyotl into American therapeutics. From time to time reports have appeared as to its efficacy in the treatment of asthma, neuralgia, rheumatism and neurasthenia.

I then asked him whether he had also taken yagé? He told me he had first learned about the devil's vine from a man called Edward Morrell Holmes, a London pharmacist and botanist. Holmes had persuaded the famous British chemist W. H. Martindale to synthesise the active alkaloid from the Banisteria vine and then offered some of the purified sample to Arthur Conan Doyle for his investigations into the spirit world.

Critchley had been intrigued by the story and had begun to carry out his own research but told me he regretted never having the opportunity to assess the liana's effect on himself. He drew my attention to an article entitled 'The Ayahuasca and Jagé Cults' that he had written in the *British Journal of Inebriety* in 1929 in which he had stated that yagé made from *Banisteria caapi* allowed the Indians to communicate with one another telepathically. The vine of the soul also imparted remote viewing faculties that enabled those who drunk it to visualise distant cities. In his article Critchley also raised the possibility that yagé might be a different plant from Banisteriopsis caapi, possibly *Prestonia amazonica*:

The pharmacological possibilities of the New World flora have as yet been investigated only superficially, but already there is ample suggestion of a wealth of untapped material.

Critchley was recognised as one of the twentieth-century giants of British neurology and his authenticity was magnetic. His restless curiosity had led him to study the sciences of anthropology and social psychology as well as the traditional teaching of his speciality and now I had learned that he had even experimented with hallucinogenic drugs. Following our chats in his home I was now even more determined to bolt down the rabbit hole in pursuit of a wonderland of distorted reality and contingent deficits.

10

– Breakthrough –

In September 1982, I sent a hand-written letter to the Secretary of the Board of Governors at the National Hospital, Queen Square, explaining that I wished to apply for the Consultant Neurologist position vacated by Doctor Gooddy. After weeks of cloak and dagger politics and whispers in the hospital corridor, news filtered down that it was going to be a close race. The informal 'trial by sherry' went well and the day after the formal inquisition, Olive Rodger, Head of the Medical Personnel department at Queen Square, called me to say I had been successful. One of my referees told me that it was my impressive list of research publications attached as an appendix to my curriculum vitae that had swung the committee in my favour. On October 5, I was appointed to the staff at both 'The National' and University College Hospitals. My new job offered me an unprecedented opportunity to pursue my research in Parkinson's disease.

Most of the patients I was still following in the clinic at University College Hospital had continued to benefit substantially from L-DOPA but the stable response that had been present in the first few years had now given way to a terrifying multidimensional rollercoaster ride that had only been temporarily slowed by the introduction of bromocriptine and deprenil. I was now confronted in the clinic with some of the most dramatic and abrupt physical transformations ever witnessed in neurological practice.

Just before Christmas I received a letter from a brave man in his sixties describing his current predicament:

It is in fact difficult now to stick to the 2-hour regime because of this apparent unreliability. If for instance I find myself 'over', suffering from so-called involuntary movements, my limbs behaving as if controlled by a drunken marionette master, I am reluctant to take a pill. So I postpone it. And then before I know where I am I am 'off'. 'On' is quite simply normal; I can survive a dinner party, drive a car, write a fair, round hand, my voice is normal. I can fall asleep rather easily unless I am trying not to. 'Off' on the other hand is very unpleasant. I lose almost all motor power in my legs; and this paralysis increasingly now spreads to my arms. Sometimes odd pains and cramps move round the body. There is no position in which I am comfortable. I can't write, I can't type, my speech is slurred and low powered. The 'off' comes on with increasingly little warning. One can adopt strategies to save oneself from various kinds of embarrassment; I have a radio taxi account to rescue me when my batteries begin to run down or if one goes 'off' suddenly in the street one holds on to a lamp post until a taxi comes past. People are extraordinarily sympathetic and helpful. I find an aluminium walking stick useful as it is a sign that something is wrong and holding on to a lamppost does not mean I am drunk. I find my 'offs' are accompanied by a curiously deep and malevolent depression. It isn't suicidal; I actually feel as if I am dying. Almost as bad is the boredom and the frustration of not being able to work. I find I am tetchy and intolerant and that it is difficult not to be bitter and sarcastic.

When I met him in the New Year he was 'off' and as he walked into my room in the outpatient clinic, he took smaller and smaller and faster and faster steps until he stumbled to the ground before I could get up and break his fall. He was a Jack-in-the-Box waiting to burst forth, still stepping internally but diminished and confined within an infinite, closed space that allowed no exit. When his L-DOPA kicked in, he orbited a Möbius strip that shot him into a hyperkinetic stratosphere only for gravitational forces to pull him back into quaking immobility. He told me his only chance was to keep moving and try to outrun the disease. A morpho fluttering its wings in Santarém or a migration of jabirus over the Pantanal had the ability to alter his uncontrollable anchored trajectory. Everything was unexpected, nothing could be relied upon.

Many of my colleagues felt that these 'on-off' swings were untreatable. The chronic bombardment of the receptors over many years from L-DOPA had led to dopamine 'burn out' and lack of responsiveness. In their view the combination of 'pharmacological blockade' with a relentless dying back of the nerve terminals, indicated that disabling fluctuations in performance were an inevitable and irremediable consequence of treatment.

My experience with the postencephalitic patients at the Highlands Hospital had convinced me that it was possible to override the slowness of movement that characterised all parkinsonian states and was now marring the long-term response to L-DOPA. 'Puskás', the football-juggling patient, had used visual cues and motor tricks to propel himself forward but one of the other patients I had seen at Highlands Hospital who was still using L-DOPA had found that he could switch back 'on' if he smoked a cigarette. Neurologists had been accused of a nihilistic scepticism towards therapies throughout my training and now that I was in a position of power I was determined to try to do everything I could to refute this unfair accusation.

I now had my first research fellow, Richard Hardie, and the two of us sat down to devise experiments that would prove to the pessimists who considered L-DOPA to be more of a curse than a cure that they were mistaken.

A group of patients, most of whom were under the age of sixty and were now experiencing severe and prolonged 'switch-offs', were selected for the first studies. On admission to hospital all tablets they were taking for Parkinson's disease were stopped and replaced by an intravenous saline infusion containing L-DOPA.

Most of the volunteers had been on treatment for more than ten years and they were now forced to carry out all their essential everyday chores during their steadily shrinking islands of mobility. The dose of L-DOPA administered through the drip was slowly increased until they 'switched on' and was then maintained uninterrupted at this steady level for the next 72 hours. During this three day awakening, some of the volunteers told us that it was like going back to the early days of L-DOPA therapy. Instead of five or six hours of mobility, the infusion had provided them with fourteen good waking hours.

The blood levels of DOPA were much more constant than those we had taken before the infusion had been started. Delayed emptying of the stomach and erratic absorption of L-DOPA tablets in the small intestine had led to peaks and troughs that had contributed to the loss of effectiveness of treatment over time. We concluded that the unconstant handling of L-DOPA in the gut and at the blood-brain barrier played a considerable part in the 'on-off phenomenon'. L-DOPA was very acidic and damaged veins, and the apparatus needed to infuse the amino acid was far too cumbersome for long term treatment, so the next step in trying to eradicate the highs and lows was to find a more viable way of continuously stimulating the dopamine system.

After a gap of too many years I was happy to be back swimming with the alkaloids, marvelling at their asymmetries adorned with rich chiral centres and decorated with dangling green heterocyclic quinolines. These intricate cyclic molecules were responsible for Nature's exquisite colours, aromatic odours and distinct tastes, and I derived pleasure from drawing their formulae on scraps of paper. Sometimes in my dreams I was in the belly of a whale, watching three dimensional vibrating plankton glide by. One night sitting on the sea bed with a telescope, a diatom with a familiar benzene ring and two hydroxyl groups and a rigid side chain supported by three carbon rings, unfurled before my eyes. This was apomorphine and I was convinced it had appeared as a direct consequence of my re-reading of *Naked Lunch* in the weeks after I had been appointed a Consultant Neurologist. William Burroughs had enthused about the drug as a cure for drug dependence, and passages in 'Deposition: Testimony Concerning a Sickness' that I had glossed over on the first reading as a medical student, now seemed to have far more importance:

The apomorphine cure is qualitatively different from other methods of cure. I have tried them all. Short reduction, slow reduction, cortisone, antihistamines, tranquilizers, sleeping cures, tolserol, reserpine. None of these cures lasted beyond the first opportunity to relapse. I can say that I was never metabolically cured until I took the apomorphine cure.
    – *Naked Lunch*

Two British chemists working at St Bartholomew's

Hospital in London in 1869 had first made apomorphine by a simple process in which opium was mixed with concentrated hydrochloric acid and then heated to 150 degrees Celsius. Shortly after the new molecule's synthesis, Samuel Gee, a physician who had trained at University College Hospital, injected two grains of the new substance into a dog, which caused it to vomit and then course the room in a peculiar repetitive way. After this, apomorphine started to be used by veterinary surgeons to treat the behavioural vices of horses, pigs and sheep.

Throughout the first half of the nineteenth century the drug was widely employed in medical practice as an emetic to expel poisons. In order to give herself a cast iron alibi, Nurse Hopkins in Agatha Christie's first Poirot novel *Sad Cypress*, injects herself with apomorphine to ensure she vomits up the tea that she had drunk from the same pot she had laced with morphia in order to poison her wealthy charge. Apomorphine was also used as an aversive therapy for the treatment of sexual deviation and alcoholism. At the end of the nineteenth century it was used at my hospital for the treatment of pseudoseizures, and for the control of St Vitus's dance (Sydenham's chorea).

In 1951, Robert Schwab, a neurologist working at the Massachusetts General Hospital in Boston, gave apomorphine to patients with Parkinson's disease on little more than a scientific hunch and reported improvement in their shakes and stiffness. Unfortunately,

the rest of the medical profession remained unenthu-
siastic about Schwab's encouraging preliminary findings although he continued to treat some of his own
patients in Boston with the drug for one or two years.
Dopamine was still of little interest to scientists, and
patients would have to wait another seventeen years
for the arrival of L-DOPA.

Apomorphine's molecular structure was much later
found to closely resemble dopamine and on this basis
it was predicted that it might be a powerful stimulator
of dopamine receptors. Parallels were also drawn between its conformational structure and that of lysergic
acid diethylamide (LSD-25).

Almost twenty years later, and now armed with a
scientific rationale denied to Schwab, George Cotzias,
working at the Brookhaven Laboratories in New Jersey,
re-examined the effect of apomorphine in Parkinson's
disease. In a series of clinical experiments conducted in
1970, he confirmed apomorphine's therapeutic potential
and felt that it might also reduce the side effects of involuntary movements and psychosis seen with L-DOPA.

Unfortunately, a lingering concern in the United
States that it might be a narcotic, the need for it to be injected, and the easy availability of L-DOPA meant that
Cotzias's findings were not followed through. There
seemed to be no place in modern neurotherapeutics for
'a nineteenth century injection that caused vomiting'.

A few weeks after my dream, I met a colleague and
friend called Eduardo Tolosa at a medical meeting and

explained to him what I now wanted to do. To convince sceptics I needed to find a rapidly acting drug that would effectively stimulate dopamine receptors so that I could follow up our experiments with infusions of L-DOPA and prove conclusively that the 'highs and lows' could be reversed by an improved delivery of dopamine to the brain. During his research fellowship, Eduardo had worked with Cotzias at Brookhaven and without hesitation he said, 'Why not try apomorphine?' The apomorphine dream of a few weeks earlier now had support from a respected colleague.

By the time of our new research studies, not a single pharmaceutical company was marketing apomorphine in the United Kingdom. After a lot of asking about, I tracked down a source of the drug suitable for human consumption. For reasons I can no longer recall, the pharmacy at the Royal Marsden Hospital on the Brompton Road had continued to manufacture supplies. One day, fifty small vials each containing two millilitres of colourless liquid arrived at the neurology office at University College Hospital.

On leaving work I took one of them home and jabbed myself with one milligram. Within a few minutes I started to feel pleasantly relaxed. I did not feel sick and the mild sedative effects disappeared in half an hour. One unexpected effect was a strong penile erection lasting about ten minutes. Only a green stain on my white shirtsleeve from a few spilled drops remained as a testimony to this first dummy run. None the worse for my experiment I returned to editing a paper Hardie had drafted and that we were keen to submit that week for publication.

After clearing it with the hospital ethics committee, we then proceeded to administer apomorphine to a group of patient volunteers during their predicted 'off' periods of DOPA unresponsiveness. Some needed reassurance that the drug was not addictive like morphine, but as in my earlier trials there was no shortage of volunteers. The long history of apomorphine use in clinical practice and my own experiment had left me in no doubt that it was safe to use.

The effects were spectacular. Every single patient was unlocked after about ten minutes and the beneficial effects of apomorphine were sustained for about an hour. A group of helpless invalids had sprung back to life and could now laugh, talk and stride effortlessly around the ward. Their 'release' reminded me of the more gradual but equally astonishing revival I had witnessed in the ticket collector who had been given L-DOPA in 1970. Hardie and I now had further evidence that the dopamine receptors in Parkinson's disease had not lost their ability to light up, despite the unnatural pounding they had received from L-DOPA. We felt increasingly confident that the on-off syndrome could be defeated by pharmacological intervention.

Apomorphine was now centre stage in my ongoing research. The relief experienced by the patient volunteers after its injection had been far more powerful than anything I had witnessed with either bromocriptine or deprenil. Gerald Stern, my senior colleague, then told me that during his National Service in the Royal Navy he had used apomorphine as an aversion therapy in a despairing chain smoker. In reply I told Gerald that I had first encountered it as the 'junk vaccine' in William Burroughs' book *Naked Lunch*. He smiled benevolently and I was secretly relieved that he had no idea what I was talking about. Medicine was still a very restrained profession. In the ensuing weeks I turned again to *Naked Lunch* and re-read 'Deposition: Testimony concerning a sickness':

The doctor explained to me that apomorphine acts on the back brain to regulate the metabolism and normalize the blood stream in such a way that the enzyme system of addiction is destroyed over a period of four or five days. Once the back brain is regulated apomorphine can be discontinued and only used in case of relapse. (No one would take apomorphine for kicks. Not one case of addiction to apomorphine has ever been recorded).

Around the same time we were carrying out the studies with apomorphine, another drug called domperidone became available that would prevent nausea and vomiting by selectively blocking dopamine receptors in a small region in the hindbrain, which acts as a sensor for the detection of noxious substances. More sophisticated portable pump delivery systems had also just become available. This technological advance would allow me to deliver apomorphine continuously through a small needle inserted under the skin of the abdominal wall. The final decisive step came when I was able to obtain financial support to employ a research nurse specifically to work on the apomorphine programme.

The first two patient volunteers were young women who had courageously lived with deadness and a creeping powerlessness for the last five years. They seesawed several times a day between an upbeat, uncoordinated jerkiness and a weighed down weakness. Their switch-offs were unpredictable, making it impossible for them to plan ahead and there was never an equipoise. The interminable twirling that came as a blessed relief to the patients in their brief windows of drug responsiveness were even more distressing for their family to behold than their debilitating stasis. They had not lost their fight or their sense of humour but their existence had become wretched and their affliction had begun to put a heavy strain on their devoted partners.

After their oscillations had been recorded and quantified in hospital, both women were started on domperidone. Two days later we began the infusion of apomorphine at a very low dose and then gradually increased the setting on the pump until they 'switched on'. It was apparent almost immediately that apomorphine was going to bring them back to life and that it would be possible to cut back on their

L-DOPA. Within a few weeks in hospital their lifeless limbs had revived and their shakes had all but gone. Their periods of incapacity had been reduced from ten hours a day to two. They had been freed from the tyranny of Parkinson's disease and could now discard their wheelchairs. The clock had been turned back on the malady by at least five years.

The miraculous improvements seen with apomorphine in Hilary B. and Liz D. and then in seventeen other severely disabled patients were described in *The Lancet* where we included a figure showing a representative 'on-off' diary to illustrate the magnitude of the improvement. Several other research groups in England and other parts of Europe confirmed our findings and within a relatively short time Burroughs' 'junk vaccine' had been rebranded as *Apo-go*, a powerful remedy for the complications of advanced Parkinson's disease. We concluded our paper with unprecedented optimism:

In general our results have been so encouraging that we would recommend that all patients seriously disabled with refractory on-off oscillations should be offered a trial of subcutaneous apomorphine, certainly before consideration of a foetal implant procedure with its attendant hazards and uncertain benefits.

The drug that had rescued Burroughs from 'The Sickness' had come to the aid of a group of desperate individuals with the shaking palsy. I will never be

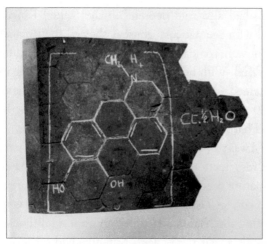

The structural formula of apomorphine on a pavement, probably drawn by Ian Sommerville in 1966. Photograph by William Burroughs.

sure how much my belief in its awakening potential stemmed directly from *Naked Lunch*.

Despite its unassailable efficacy, apomorphine failed to capture the public imagination or interest the scientific press. The implantation of foetal dopamine cells in Sweden filled the papers, even though the approach was unproven and only four people had been treated so far, without improvement. My only concern now was that I could continue to use apomorphine to treat my patients and that this fantastic 'oldie but goodie' would be made available to the thousands of patients who were turning once more to ice. I contacted the small family business of Britannia Pharmaceuticals who had also sold deprenil in the United Kingdom and with the patients' consent showed their management team some of the videos we had recorded during the trial. With help from Gerald Stern and I, the firm obtained a licence from the Medicines Agency and in 1993 apomorphine returned triumphantly to the British Pharmacopoeia.

I was pleased that I had played an important part in the resurrection of a disregarded treatment. However, a 'mature product' that was simple to manufacture and had cost us just a few pounds to investigate was now costing the National Health Service several thousand pounds a year per patient. Britannia had successfully made the case to the authorities that apomorphine was a Rolls Royce drug that had been previously undersold for the price of a bicycle! In the first few years after the company had obtained a licence, it made great efforts to ensure quality control and close down a number of 'illicit distilleries' – National Health Service pharmacies who were making the drug at a cut rate and eating away at their business model. I understood the need to be profitable and was grateful to Britannia for making apomorphine available but I felt uncomfortable about a system where money was made out of illness and where the patient was treated as a customer. The company knew the price but not the value to the patients. I made it clear I was not for hire and that I wanted no shares or financial interest in the firm.

11

– The Junk Vaccine –

After we had been using apomorphine for about a year, I was contacted by Ann Langford Dent, the daughter of John Yerbury Dent, the physician who had treated William Burroughs in London for narcotic addiction. She, along with her elder sister, Jane Yerbury Sweeney, had continued to hold a torch for their father's treatment methods and hoped that I could join their life-long campaign to encourage psychiatrists to re-evaluate apomorphine's efficacy as a healthier more effective alternative to methadone. In one of her distinctive handwritten letters distinguished by her large attractive script and headed with an eye-catching ink drawing of the human herd on the Kings Road, Ann wrote:

Grandchild No.6 aged four months and a commission to paint a mural 10 feet by 10 feet keep me busy, but as I can see the light at the end of the tunnel my crowning satisfaction would be to see Apomorphine used to cure alcoholics and drug addicts.

In the spring of 1956, William Burroughs had travelled from the native quarter of Tangier to England. His dependence on synthetic opioids had become so

absolute that he had not removed his clothes for almost a year except to stick a needle into his fibrous,
sallow skin:

I am not an addict I am the addict. The addict I invented to
keep this show on the junk road. I am all the addicts and all
the junk in the world. I am junk and I am hooked for ever.
  – *The Beginning is also the End*

His distraught parents had paid for his flight to
England and arranged for a referral to a Dr MacClay
in Queens Gate Place. MacClay did not see Burroughs
but referred him directly to his Kensington colleague,
Dr Dent, a practitioner who had gained a reputation
for the treatment of chronic anxiety and alcohol dependence. Dent had summarised his views in a best-
selling book entitled *Anxiety and its Treatment with
Special Reference to Alcoholism* (1941), in which he
provided convincing and measured arguments that the
chronically anxious were at particular risk of developing serious addictions. Despite his distaste for public
office and complete absence of political nous, he had
also served dutifully as the Secretary of *The Society for
the Study of Addiction* from 1944 to 1947.

After qualification at Kings College Hospital in
London, Dent worked for five years at the St Pancras
South Infirmary, where he had learned to use apomorphine injections to sober up stuporous drunks brought
in by the police. In an oral presentation delivered

before The Society for the Study of Addiction in 1948, he recanted his earlier view that apomorphine was an aversion therapy. Based on his extensive experience in more than two hundred and fifty alcoholics he told the Society's members that apomorphine worked through a specific 'metabolic' action on the 'sleep centre' in the hindbrain. Morphine and alcohol inhibited the fore-brain whereas apomorphine stimulated the back brain and particularly the almond-sized hypothalamus.

Dent was a contradictory character, gracious yet brusque, argumentative, shy yet noisy but smart enough to know that shit happens on a daily basis in medicine without any help from arrogance, vanity or incompetence. One acquaintance likened him to an intellectual Brigadier-General. He was fortunate to practice in an intrepid era where doctors were allowed to treat patients based on their own conscience and openly challenge dogma without risk of being struck off the medical register. Dent enjoyed his autonomy and was free to prescribe what he liked. He didn't need guidelines from so-called experts but based his decision making on his experience and knowledge. Although he was an atheist, the Quaker principles of his family – simplicity, pacifism, integrity, community and equality (SPICE) defined his medical ethics. His practice was run on Robin Hood lines; the rich were expected to pay more to subsidise his poorer patients. In a post-war world of back street abortion, gay sex crime and the continuing shame of intemperance, he was one of the few who had the courage to treat the forsaken and disheartened. He was also a consultant at St Mary's Ursuline Convent in Surrey where the nuns took in women addicts and treated them with great success under Dent's guidance.

A few months before Burroughs arrived on his doorstep, Dent had written an editorial in the October 1955 edition of the *British Journal of Addiction (Alcohol and Other Drugs)* condemning the British Government's recent decision to stop the legal production of heroin in the UK. He warned that a flourishing black market in narcotics was now inevitable and despaired that the State was even more ignorant than the medical profession about the mechanisms of addiction. A few months earlier he had also written to the *Journal of the American Medical Association* regretting the lack of enthusiasm for apomorphine in the United States. He believed that maintenance treatment was trading one addiction for another and conforming to an economic imperative. Hundreds of deaths were occurring every year from methadone overdose. It was the perfect capitalist scam.

34 Addison Road was a large comfortable house separated from the road by a stuccoed stone wall with a kennel at the front for Dent's Scottish terrier. The first floor had been modified to accommodate his surgery and a small receptionist's office and had a fine view onto a pretty but unkempt English garden with a fish-pond and a random sprinkling of creepers and shrubs.

Burroughs, dressed in a sombre grey suit, rang the

doorbell and waited nervously with hat in hand, fearing the doctor might turn him over to 'the heat'. Dent opened the door in his braces, a stocky short man with shaggy white hair and a moustache. Over a cup of tea in front of a blazing fire, he tried to relax his new patient with a few light-hearted asides. Burroughs told Dent that from the age of thirty he had seldom been sober although he had not always been addicted to drugs, that he had taken ten cures and after every one he had lapsed at the first opportunity. An episode of delirium in Tangier had freaked him out and made him realise that if he didn't come off dope immediately he would soon be dead. To his surprise, Dent then asked him if he would feel more comfortable if he had an injection of morphine, to which Burroughs replied, 'Well that would help.'

Burroughs went on to tell Dent that before leaving Tangier he had been hitting with methadone every hour, using up to 15 grains a day. At this point Dent got up to feed his tropical fish. By the time the doctor sat down again he had come to the conclusion that Burroughs was a hard-boiled American who genuinely wanted to quit narcotics but would not be taken in by any form of pompous medical bullshit. Dent explained that he was not a moralist but a chemist and that chronic opiate use had caused a metabolic dysregulation in Burroughs' brainstem. Although apomorphine treatment should be continued for no longer than ten days, remission could not be considered to have occurred until a month after that. He also warned him that the treatment could be unpleasant, particularly during the first two days. Sixty per cent of the patients he had treated with apomorphine had managed to remain off alcohol or drugs.

He also informed Burroughs that according to the Home Office there were only 306 people addicted in Britain to opium, heroin, morphine and Indian hemp. Just under half of these were women and over half of the male addicts were physicians. As Burroughs got up to leave, Dent informed him that he wanted him to switch from methadone to morphine prior to apomorphine, to which Burroughs replied, 'Magnificent man.'

Burroughs was admitted to 99 Cromwell Road, a four-storey building that also housed an abortion clinic. He had his own room with rose-coloured wallpaper and round-the-clock personal nursing care from Sister Morse and Sister Gibson, Dent's two nurses. Apomorphine was injected in a dose of one twentieth of a grain every two hours day and night, gradually increasing the interval between injections. He was advised to remain in bed and was prescribed Vitamin B supplements and was also allowed to take diminishing quantities of morphine over the first three days. On one occasion, Dent arrived unannounced at two in the morning and stayed talking to the wide-awake Burroughs until dawn. Dent knew that addiction had a huge psychological dimension and that any method used to convince a patient into adapting to a differing strategy for life needed to be holistic. Burroughs experienced far fewer withdrawal symptoms with apomorphine than with any of the other detoxification treatment approaches he had tried. He slept very little but the slow, painful, constricting feeling of death that he had come to associate with opiate withdrawal was absent.

On discharge from the clinic he was given some tubes of apomorphine pellets to use in the event of delayed withdrawal symptoms and instructed to stay at his lodgings at 44 Egerton Gardens for the next seven days. Dent visited him there and re-emphasised to his patient that he would need to reach a state of mind in the ensuing months where he no longer wanted narcotics. He pointed out that apomorphine was an effective treatment but the onus of travelling beyond a tomorrow free of pain and junk lay firmly on Burroughs' shoulders. Dent used his considerable motivating powers to encourage his patient to stick at writing as a form of therapy and also recommended that he follow up with some complementary therapy including an abdominal exercise system. In Dent's view there was no such thing as willpower when it came to addiction.

Burroughs' attitude to doctors was ambiguous. He equated the paternalism of the doctor-patient relationship with the dependency of the addict on his pusher. Medical practitioners were the opium of the people. Many 'croakers' as he referred to doctors, were greedy, corrupt and ineffectual and some exerted damaging nocebo effects on their trusting patients. His creation of the amoral Benway was his revenge for the corruption that he felt defined doctoring. Burroughs was medicine's nemesis and a living Doctor Benway. At the same time he longed for a physician who could help him obliterate his ruminant viral fears and become a trusted ally.

Burroughs described Dr Dent as the least paranoid of men, and a physician who possessed 'the full warmth and goodwill the English were able to offer'. He was the nearest thing Burroughs ever had to a Dr Watson. Their ideas were uncannily similar, and their relationship more like father and son than doctor and patient. When the two had first met, both were at the end of the line. Burroughs was addicted to drugs and unable to write, Dent was dying of consumption and had been denigrated by his profession as a maverick. Both men were iconoclasts who held a distaste for globalisation and consumerism and shared an affection for cats.

They exchanged stories and discussed subjects of mutual interest. Burroughs warmed to his doctor's loud laugh and confident professional approach. Dent reinforced to Burroughs that he had great potential as a writer. By today's standards his stewardship of Burroughs might have been censured by the General Medical Council but at that time the profession was more preoccupied with breaches of confidentiality and the misdemeanour of advertising than curbing the freedoms of the doctor-patient dynamic. Dent was not the only one promoting the use of apomorphine. There were similar champions in France, Switzerland and Denmark, all reporting good results in private practice.

In a letter to Allen Ginsberg on May 8 1956, Burroughs described his experience with 'Dent's cure' as unpleasant but nowhere near as bad as some of his previous detox experiences and that he was now determined to make it. He also commented on the pleasantly relaxing effect of apomorphine. In a second letter posted a week later he stated that he was now fully recovered, no longer dwelling on his previous way of life and that he was able to drink alcohol again. He hated the grim greyness ('London drags like an anchor') and headed back to Tangier from where he wrote yet again to Ginsberg informing him that he had completely lost all desire for narcotics and sex.

Encouraged by Dent, Burroughs wrote 'Letter from a Master Addict to Dangerous Drugs', which would be published in *The British Journal of Addiction* (Volume 53, issue no 2, 1957). In this article, written for medical practitioners, Burroughs stated he had become an addict because he did not have strong motivations in any other direction. He was bored and disillusioned after Harvard and didn't know what to do with his life. He had first taken junk out of curiosity. He had then drifted through life taking shots whenever he could score, attracted by the outlaw lifestyle and the glamour of gangsterhood. He had never wanted to be an addict but one day he woke up feeling sick and realised he was hooked. He went on to say that apomorphine was by far the best method of treating withdrawal he had experienced in that it reduced the symptoms to an endurable level and led to a more rapid recovery than any reduction cure. Apomorphine had abolished the craving and almost certainly saved his life. In Burroughs' words, saying an addict had been cured by methadone was like saying an alcoholic had been cured of whisky by the use of gin.

This watered-down article pigeonholed him as a biased addict whose evidence could not be relied upon and was greeted with disdain by Dent's medical opponents.

Despite Burroughs' claim that 'the junk vaccine' could evict the addict personality, it was not a permanent cure for his habit. In the first few years after his 'cure' he relapsed twice on a French compound containing opium called *Eubispasme Codethyline* and needed further visits to Dent and courses of apomorphine pellets to get himself straightened out. For several years he carried a supply of apomorphine with him wherever he went as a preventative.

On 27 July 1960, Burroughs wrote to Dent from The Empress Hotel, 25 Lillie Road, London:

Dear Doctor Dent

I don't know if Harry Phipps told you about my intention to write an article on a popular level concerning the apomorphine treatment of all addictions. I hope you will give me permission to quote from your book . . .

– *Rub Out the Words: Letters 1959–1974*

A year later Dent wrote to Burroughs:

Dear Burroughs,

Thank you very much for the Naked Lunch which arrived safely. I congratulate you on it. I do sympathise with you on your country's idiocy in its attitude to apomorphine we shall win in the end . . .

Yours as ever

J. Dent

On January 16 1962, Rhoda Brennan, a close friend who had lived with her husband and Dent at Addison Road, wrote to Burroughs from 160 Holland Park Avenue, London:

Dear Mr Burroughs

I know you will be sad to hear that John Dent died very suddenly on Jan 8th. It was a coronary thrombosis and he died as he would have liked sitting in his chair in the dining room playing patience . . .

He was so fond of you and interested in your work. I wish there was any one like him to carry on his work but I'm afraid there isn't.

Yours sincerely

Rhoda Brennan

For Dent, apomorphine was always work in progress and after his death William Burroughs became his standard bearer, railing against the US Narcotics Bureau, and the American Medical Association's refusal to condone the treatment. In Burroughs' opinion addicts should never be asked the question 'Why did you start using narcotics in the first place?' It was as irrelevant as asking a man with blackwater fever why he had travelled to a malarial infested region. He felt that reliving the addict experience as a form of therapy was positively dangerous and that psycho-analysis should be contra-indicated.

In a panel debate organised by *Playboy* magazine in New York in 1970, which included the veteran Commissioner of the Bureau of Narcotics, Harry J. Anslinger, and John Finlator, Director of the Food and Drug Administration's Bureau of Drug Abuse Control, Burroughs was asked his views on how the problem of heroin addiction could be controlled:

Apomorphine is listed in the United States as a narcotic sub-ject to the same regulations as morphine but in both France and England only an ordinary prescription is required and it can be refilled any number of times. Its difficult to avoid the conclusion that a deliberate attempt has been made in the United States to mislead medical opinion and minimize the value of this treatment.

Throughout the second half of the twentieth cen-tury the use of heroin in the United Kingdom slowly increased and became a degrading lonely lifestyle choice for large numbers of young men. People no longer became addicts by chance as perhaps they had in Burroughs' day. In the deprived inner cities 'trains-potting' and 'dragon chasing' was a salient part of life for increasing numbers of clueless losers with time on their hands.

By the eighties, scientific evidence had accrued in support of Dent's views but ironically apomorphine's use had slowly fizzled out. Burroughs was finding it increasingly difficult to recommend physicians who were prepared to provide apomorphine for his many addicted correspondents. Mrs Smith ('Smitty'), one of Dent's old nurses now living over a pub in Devon, was still giving apomorphine and had treated Keith Richards in his Cheyne Walk apartment. In his autobiography, the Rolling Stone guitarist described 'Smitty' as vicious and authoritarian, and apomorphine as aversive – the worst torture he had ever experienced. Perhaps the molecule's great antiquity with its chequered history as a sedative, expectorant and emetic had something to do with it. Its name had also counted against it with the public.

In July 1983, Burroughs wrote to Isabelle Aubert-Baudron, curator of the *Interzone*, a web-based French publishing house, expressing his frustration over the attitude of doctors and the imminent demise of apomorphine:

Doctors are, by and large drastically limited in outlook. They have read all there is to know on any subject and that is that. Anything outside their knowledge cannot be worth hearing about. So I really gave up years ago. Some doctors in Denmark still use the apo treatment but they clash with the psychiatrists. In my opinion a substantial number of psychiatrists should be broken down to veterinarians but that goes for the medical profession in general.

Fully acquainted with the scientific facts, I now supported Dent's daughters' campaign to get the medical establishment to re-investigate the apomorphine pump as a treatment for heroin and alcohol dependence, but my pleas fell on deaf ears. Big Pharma were not interested in drug addiction because of the inherent risks involved. One of the concerns was that even if a new treatment showed promising results an addict might simply override his treatment by overdosing on opiates, leading to bad publicity for their product. The addiction specialists I contacted either failed to respond or said they were too busy to consider setting up a trial. I got the feeling a self-perpetuating substance dependence industry had grown up with strong survival instincts and ambitions for further expansion.

After our seminal publication in 1988, apomorphine's use for the treatment of Parkinson's disease had rapidly spread round the world yet despite its undisputed effectiveness it had not yet managed to clear the regulators in the United States. It had run into the same brick wall Dent had experienced thirty years earlier.

Throughout the 1990s I carried out many clinical pharmacological experiments to better understand apomorphine's mode of action and find ways of avoiding the need for injections. Large numbers of morphine derivatives were flooding the market and being dished out to excess in the treatment of chronic pain but the pharmaceutical industry showed no interest in clinical trials on the related aporphines for the management of neurological and psychiatric disorders. Apomorphine survived as an expensive and underused 'orphan drug' treatment. At times of disappointment, Burroughs' writing spurred me on:

No doubt substances fifty times stronger than apomorphine could be developed and the side effect of vomiting eliminated . . . I suggest that research with variations of apomorphine and synthesis of it will open a new frontier extending far beyond the problem of addiction.
– *Naked Lunch*

Groups of atoms with structures closely related to apomorphine had now been identified in the flowers and tubers of the Maya's sacred water lilies and I felt that their study might offer an interesting alternative to Burroughs' scientific suggestion of spinning the molecular roulette wheel. I was still drawn to the idea that the cure for Parkinson's disease might lie hidden deep in the Amazon forest and that the chemical structures of lianas, roots and barks might serve as templates from which drug compounds could be created.

12

– Hooked on the Medicine –

I n 1999, completely out of the blue, the wife of
one of my patients told me that apomorphine had
turned her husband into a junky. Over the last year he
had become infatuated with its 'cloud nine' effects and
he had lost all interest in her and the rest of his family. He binged on food, spent money irresponsibly and
acted out fantasies with a sex therapist. Sometimes he
disappeared for hours and was brought home late at
night by the police or paramedics who suspected he
was 'crack dancing'.

Mr C denied most of his wife's story but admitted
that over the last year he had developed a deep fear of
the doom he associated with medication 'switch-offs'.
He also conceded that after taking an L-DOPA cap-
sule or an injection of apomorphine he sometimes felt
like a world-beater. I explained to both of them that
to my knowledge craving for apomorphine had never
been reported in the medical literature. I instructed
the patient to limit the number of 'rescue' shots he was
giving himself to a maximum of six a day and to cut
back a little on his L-DOPA.

Not long after I had dismissed out of hand the
possibility of addiction to apomorphine, a second,

equally concerning story was drawn to my attention, (a train of events well recognised in medicine that frequently marks the first step in the delineation of a new syndrome). A commercial salesman whom I had been treating for four years told me that over the last few months he had felt an uncontrollable drive to take more and more L-DOPA even though he realised that he may be overdosing. In the space of a year he had doubled his dose and still was not satisfied with the effect. Later that afternoon, I re-read the chastening letter I had received from Mr C's wife a week after the fraught consultation:

Dear Dr Lees,

My husband has changed fundamentally. He has become obsessed with his drugs, their administration, and particularly their effects on his physical condition. It is now like living with a horrible stranger. He has started to lie to me about every-thing. He never lied before. He has become financially extrav-agant, so much so that we are now in a great deal of debt. He was always careful and responsible about money. He is inject-ing himself 15 times a day over his prescribed dose and always has a pocket full of L-DOPA. As for our sexual partnership, that stopped when he discovered that 'Planet Apomorphine' was better than sex. I was secretly pleased, as I was so angry I wouldn't have sex with him anyway. He is no longer the man I married. He has also recently developed 'fantasy attachments' to old girlfriends and to some of my female friends and has started to act out his fantasies either by harassing them, turn-ing up at their door late at night in an agitated state or, more

frequently, endlessly telephoning them. At the recent consultation, I felt as if I was seen as the 'problem' and that you
did not believe me. I hope that after receiving this letter you
will consider admitting my husband to hospital for a period
of detoxification.

I now understood that I had remained too focused
on relieving the patient's physical discomfort and been
oblivious to the undesirable consequences of his medication. I questioned whether my keenness for apomorphine that had returned to neurological practice six
years earlier, had clouded my judgement. I had been
guilty of blinkered thinking but was still not sure that I
needed to apologise. Abuse of medicines prescribed by
doctors for pain and mental illness was well recognised
but the notion that a highly effective treatment for a
degenerative neurological disorder could cause a damaging chemical dependency still seemed implausible.

Gavin Giovannoni, my senior registrar, and I subsequently identified a further thirteen individuals, all
of whom complained that despite a massive escalation
of their L-DOPA dose their medication was becoming
less and less effective. These patients could sometimes
be recognised in the outpatient waiting room because
of their drug-fuelled gyrating whirls and pirouettes
and their total inability to sit still. They stood out from
the motionless silent majority by their restless pacing
and fidgeting. When they entered the consulting room
they complained bitterly of being 'under pilled'. They

had pressured speech, seemed to be distracted and were hard to engage in rational conversation. Some were drenched in sweat and unable to concentrate.

One young man told me he had become a slave to his medication and had started to visit other doctors' surgeries asking for supplies of L-DOPA. I thought of Burroughs' advice to junkies, 'You need a good bedside manner with doctors or you will get nowhere'. One of the patients who I had admitted to the hospital in an attempt to reduce his medication confided in me later that he had left his car close to the hospital in a long stay car park and had sneaked out regularly without the nurses' knowledge to take extra L-DOPA from a cache stockpiled in the boot of his car.

We soon realised that these 'overusing' patients frequently had very disturbed behaviour patterns that included morbid jealousy (the Othello syndrome), irresponsible ruinous internet and scratch card betting and hypersexuality. Unbeknown to his wife, one man had ordered twenty four pet Mexican turtles that arrived at his home by courier, while another man went to the supermarket for a loaf of bread and returned with ten romantic DVDs. One man in his fifties had been imprisoned for attempted rape and another had given away thousands of pounds to a stranger in a bout of reckless generosity. In some cases the seriousness of the medication dependency had only come to light during emergency hospital admissions when the nurses reported to the medical staff that the patient was constantly demanding extra pills. A sense of shame and profound embarrassment combined with a reluctance to associate the damaging behaviour to their medical lifeline had driven a grave problem under the surface. Two of the wives had filed for divorce because of their husband's insatiable sexual demands. During our investigations I received another desperate letter from a patient's wife:

I am pretty much at the end of the line now. My husband is acting so strangely, has cut himself off from me and his daughter who he adores and is almost paranoid that people are watching him. He is living in a complete bubble and honestly thinks that we will all be fine about his selfish actions. He is holding false beliefs which cannot be changed by fact. I literally can't go on any more and for the psychiatrist to basically say he doesn't think there is anything wrong with him is beyond me.

House calls had become a vital part of our inquiries as it was only in the patients' homes that we could appreciate the true extent of the mayhem. It was also as a result of these domiciliary visits that another hidden and equally disruptive behaviour came to light. We learned that some individuals were carrying out repetitive ritualistic behaviours for hours on end at the expense of everything else, including eating and drinking. A seamstress collected and endlessly sorted thousands of buttons, while another woman withdrew into herself and spent all night marking every object in her house with yellow sticky labels. A man circled London on the orbital bypass twenty or more times a night in his car, while a retired engineer had constructed a monstrous Heath-Robinson computer that grew and grew until it filled the whole of one bedroom. A former jeweller spent all his time purposelessly dismantling old watches and putting them back together again.

These purposeless activities first reported in bikers using large amounts of intravenous amphetamine had been termed punding, a Swedish word meaning 'blockhead'. During a 'run', some of the amphetamine addicts would pound up and down the same part of the street, or march in circles, often lifting their legs high. A visitor to the Burroughs' household in New Orleans described how Joan Vollmer would spend all day washing the kitchen wall, mopping and scrubbing the floor of the children's room and sweeping lizards off the dead tree in the yard while neglecting her own personal hygiene and that of her children – classical signs of Benzedrine-induced punding.

After several rejections by high impact neurology journals it was evident that the anonymous peer reviewers were highly sceptical of our findings. Some of the comments were scathing and derogatory. One suggested that we had misinterpreted the patients' stories. The anonymous peer review system that was held in such great esteem seemed to me archaic and dishonest. It was ponderous, prone to bias and abuse and a bit of a lottery. It was also ineffective at spotting errors and deceit. If a referee for a scientific journal had concerns or criticisms about my paper then they should be prepared to release their name.

We had entitled our paper 'Hedonistic homeostatic dysregulation' – technical jargon we lifted from the substance dependence literature in the hope of reducing the risk of media sensationalism and the subsequent inevitable clamour of concern driven by ambulance chasers. 'Addict' carried moral connotations that suggested the individual was of weak will and low moral fibre. I did not want to cast doubt yet again on L-DOPA, the single most important therapeutic advance to have occurred in neurology in the previous fifty years.

A sick joke now going around the pharmaceutical industry was that in the current safety-first society of Western Europe, the most profitable drug to licence and market was a placebo. More and more effort was going into the development of 'harmless' drugs with marginal benefits. An increasingly risk-averse society was stifling innovation and I didn't want to give the lawyers any more ammunition. The *Journal of Neurology, Neurosurgery and Psychiatry* finally accepted our paper on 24 August 1999, after it had gone through two rounds of extensive but inconsequential revisions.

The idea that patients could develop an addiction to L-DOPA or apomorphine was considered fanciful and greeted with incredulity by most neurologists. Some thought we were simply describing a pathological failure to resist harmful temptations that had recently been acknowledged as an uncommon complication of therapy with dopamine agonist drugs and which I had first witnessed in the lady on bromocriptine, gambling her money away at bingo in 1976.

After I had presented our findings at an international Parkinson's disease conference, one famous and well respected neurologist stood up and stated that he had treated thousands of patients with L-DOPA over thirty years and had never encountered a patient who had become addicted to the treatment. His intonation and manner suggested that I had a vivid imagination and was irresponsibly seeking publicity. He expressed surprise that the editors of a reputable journal had published our findings and went on to say that if by any remote chance our observations had validity then they could be adequately explained by a patient's understandable attempt to avoid an aversive dysphoric dopamine withdrawal state.

Experience had taught me to expect this negative reaction to our findings. In many ways it encouraged me because it indicated we had reported something that, despite its gravity, hadn't been recognised by our colleagues. The reason the distinguished colleague who had cast doubt on our findings had not seen it could be explained by the fact that most of his patients came only once to his office and were then sent back to the referring physician. Despite the opposition within the neurological world I was now convinced of the importance of our naïve empiricism. I also now knew that I had heard similar stories several years earlier but had dismissed them out of hand.

Just before the paper describing our shocking findings was published, Oliver Sacks, who had now become a friend and occasional visitor to my department, had been moved to congratulate the Editor of *JAMA Neurology* for permitting a healthy debate in its correspondence column in relation to the lingering suggestions that L-DOPA might actually accelerate dopamine nerve cell loss. He contrasted the journal's democratic approach to the violent reaction he had faced thirty years earlier when he had drawn attention to the potential of L-DOPA to cause pathological sensitivities in postencephalitic patients. He then nailed his colours to the mast with respect to his own therapeutic preferences:

I would certainly want to be put on L-DOPA myself, if I became parkinsonian, because nothing else can give comparable benefit. I would want this even knowing that its effects would sooner or later decline and be compromised, and that it might accelerate the disease process or cause neuronal death. The immediate benefit, for me, would outweigh the incalculable future. But others might feel very differently.

Field work in which we had recorded the distressing stories of our patients' families had taken us this far but if we were to convince our dubious critics we now needed help from psychiatrists working in the field of drug dependency. Jenny Bearn from the Bethlem Addictions Unit in South London agreed to collaborate, and her research fellow, Mike Kelleher, interviewed the 'overusing' patients to determine if they fulfilled established operational psychiatric criteria for addiction. Semi-structured questionnaires were administered in order to distinguish whether adaptive therapeutic dependence on L-DOPA and apomorphine or a pathological pattern of use was responsible. Compared with the matched control patients, the 'DOPA dysregulators' experienced more euphoria on medication and more dissatisfaction during the 'switched off' state. Dopamine replacement therapy was affecting their lives negatively. One of them had used amphetamine as a stimulant for several years during his teens and two were alcoholics.

We concluded that a small sub-group of patients had become abnormally dependent on dopamine replacement therapy, a finding that not only had implications for treatment choice in Parkinson's disease, but also provided further indirect evidence for the role of dopamine in the genesis of substance dependence.

We next attempted to construct a profile of the dysregulating 'addicts' personality before the onset of their Parkinson's disease from meetings with their family. The patients were asked to fill in some personality inventories with the instruction that they must try to recall what they had been like in the years before their illness had begun, rather than how they felt now. Most of the DOPA addicts were men who had been struck down with Parkinson's disease in their thirties, forties and fifties and they exhibited risk-taking novelty-seeking traits on the tests similar to those frequently reported in alcoholics and drug addicts. Their behaviour was the converse of that seen in the large majority of people with Parkinson's disease, who tended to be introspective, cautious, anhedonic, non-smokers.

Apart from our collaborators at the Bethlem Hospital there was little initial interest in our findings from addiction specialists who rarely read neurology journals and attend different medical meetings. My earlier attempts to kindle interest in further trials with apomorphine in substance-dependence had taught me that psychiatrists were greatly constrained by government policy in relation to what trials they could carry out and what they could safely say in public. After the farrago of misinformation with deprenil I was also determined to minimise any press coverage of our findings. Nevertheless, the dopamine dysregulators offered a perfect surrogate for research into addiction.

I did receive one or two letters from psychiatrists who raised the very reasonable question that if taking L-DOPA was so rewarding why was it not being used more on the street like other dopamine drugs such as amphetamine and cocaine?

Elucidation of this conundrum came when one of my patients introduced me to a demi-monde of blogs on the grey web where neophytes recounted a candy-land dream world of DOPA 'highs.' The mere contemplation of taking a tablet was a source of great joy for one man who had managed to buy L-DOPA on the Internet. Bodybuilders described using herbal sources of the amino acid (the beans of the cowhage plant) that they had bought to increase muscle bulk and experiencing libidinous and aggressive impulses similar to those they had felt with anabolic steroids. A young sybarite had left an account of a DOPA trip in which he had experienced enhanced colour vision and a 'return to a childhood world of exceptional beauty and innocence'. On a patient chatline someone had written, 'Had an insane high on 250 mg L-DOPA, felt like I was king of the earth, sex drive way above my normal levels and feels as if it is still increasing, sensations all take longer and the feel is multiplied, fantastic dreams that are so amazingly vivid that makes it feel as if I have another world to go to when I sleep.' The patient then told me that his first 'hit' had caused a rush through the brain that had never been repeated. He extolled the virtues of Sinemet (one of the proprietary names for L-DOPA) in the following ode:

> Sinemet, Sinemet, Sinemet plus!
> We have a penchant for all things yellow
> Our favourite colour, it's oh so mellow!
> When one of us is sick or disturbed
> We just give him little yellow pills
> And in 20 seconds, he's feeling better.

I now wanted to understand more about substance abuse – a topic that I had read little about since extra-curricular reading during medical school. I started to plough through the reams of academic theorising and barely comprehensible psychobabble that had been published in medical journals. The experimental work of Berridge and Robinson, the imaging studies of Nora Volkow in cocaine addicts and Koob and Le Moal's theory of hedonistic homeostatic dysregulation were instructive but it was the unsentimental fieldwork of the arch self-experimenter, William Burroughs, that best helped me to understand DOPA abuse. I re-read *Junkie* and *Naked Lunch* and this time I paid particular attention to Burroughs' descriptions of the 'algebra of need' and the machinery of control. In a spirit of sci-entific enquiry, Burroughs had offered his neurones up as a culture medium for the junk virus. Unsentimental and factual, he wrote as if his thoughts had the quality of self-evidence:

Because there are many forms of addiction I think they will all obey basic laws. The drug addict will do *anything* to satisfy total need . . . A rabid dog cannot choose but bite. The addict of any sort has sacrificed all control, and is as dependent as an unborn child.
   – *Naked Lunch*

Burroughs often spoke of his self-hatred of the ad-dict lifestyle. He considered junk to be an analgesic that killed the pain and pleasure implicit in awareness. He quoted the British neurophysiologist Sir Charles Sherrington as stating that pain is the psychic adjunct to an imperative protective reflex. Heroin destabilised the vegetative nervous system and cut off all feeling, diminishing the addict to a passive plant-like existence. Burroughs believed addiction was neither a moral failing nor a psychiatric disorder. 'It's as psychological as malaria' he wrote.

Life telescoped down to 'fixes', anticipation of the next hit and the paraphernalia of addiction. As the junk parasite infested the body all other interests and activities lost their importance. The junky needed to score to get out of bed in the morning, to shave and eat breakfast. Junk was in some way alive and the junky was a saprophyte:

The addict runs on junk time. His body is the clock, and junk runs through it like an hourglass. Time has meaning for him only with reference to his need.
– *Naked Lunch*

Burroughs never idealised or promoted the junkie lifestyle. He was not an advocate of drug use but regarded drug addiction as a medical rather than criminal issue. Nevertheless, many heroin addicts dying in high-rise squats now regarded *Naked Lunch* as their Bible. For them he had become the bard of the decaying city.

In Burroughs opinion junk blanked out torment,

eased the passage of painful time and had the potential to protect a vulnerable individual from schizophrenia and alcoholism. Regular usage of narcotics created an irresistible, pleasureless desire at the expense of everything else. Junkies were members of a disreputable and immediately recognisable club but only accepted they were different from the herd when they ran out of dope. They were bores who went through the motions, heroin was profane.

In the Introduction of the original *Junk* manuscript I found passages that differentiated the requirement for prescribed medicines from the desire for recreational drugs:

The junkie needs junk like the diabetic needs insulin. Junk creates a deficiency so that the body cannot function without more junk at regular intervals. It seems that junk takes over the function of certain body chemicals during addiction. Withdrawal of junk creates a deficiency condition, which continues until the body gets back in production on the chemicals that were replaced by junk. When I say 'habit forming drug' I mean a drug that alters the endocrine balance of the body in such a way that the body requires that drug in order to function. So far as I know, junk is the only habit-forming drug according to this definition.

In 'Letter of a Master Addict' he distinguished the junkie from the insulin-dependent diabetic:

The diabetic will die without insulin, but he is not addicted to insulin. His need for insulin was not brought about by the use of insulin. He needs insulin to maintain a normal metabolism. The addict needs morphine to maintain a morphine metabolism, and so avoid the excruciatingly painful return to a normal metabolism.

Narcotic addiction was a drug-induced metabolic disturbance, a form of chronic poisoning that created a craving as intense as thirst and for which the only antidote was more junk.

Although the Parkinson dysregulators had been prescribed L-DOPA as a life-enhancing medicine, similar mechanisms seemed to be at work. Their medicine no longer made them feel better or well but was still badly needed. Burroughs emphasised that 'Junk is not a Kick'. L-DOPA had led to disinhibition, impaired decision-making and an escalation of medication use. Cutting the L-DOPA dose by half and restricting apomorphine had reduced the risky behaviour of the first patient but deprived him of his zip. He was more 'manageable' and more acceptable to his wife but he now complained that he felt flat and had lost all *joie de vivre*. Several months after his dependence had been brought under control he wrote me a letter:

I have stopped cross-dressing since I reduced my daily dose of dopa and find this to be much more socially acceptable. But privately I must admit that I rather miss my skirts as I used to get a blast of 'feel good factor' when I put them on, that overrode any aches and pains I may have had at that time.

Burroughs described similar feelings of hollowness and ennui when he was off junk:

Then you hit a sag. It is an effort to dress, get out of a chair, pick up a fork. You don't want to do anything or go anywhere. The junk craving is gone but there isn't anything else.

– *Junkie*

After I had managed to successfully withdraw another of the addicted patients from damagingly high doses of L-DOPA, his wife took me to one side and thanked me for returning her husband to her after two years of hell. His secretiveness, capricious moods and Jekyll and Hyde behaviour had vanished and he had returned to being the loving compassionate man she had married. She was eternally grateful for what I had done, but her husband complained to me in confidence that a dense fog had descended on his life and he had lost his 'buzz'.

Although much of Burroughs' 'word hoard' had been written in a narcotic and marijuana haze, he emphasised that junk stifled the creative urge. Apomorphine had been the turning point between life and death and without its help he would never have been able to put together the fugues from which *Naked Lunch* emerged. Freed from opioids his drive returned and with the disinfected eyes of the revived writer he could clearly visualise the Inferno.

A well-known novelist with Parkinson's disease

who I had been treating for several years told me that his literary productivity was greatly enhanced by the use of apomorphine injections and he refused to cut back despite the fact that his arms were covered in puncture marks and bruises and his continuous writing was destroying his relationship with his wife. When I asked him why he was using apomorphine at times when he was already mobile, he took a picture of his rose garden out of his pocket and turned to me, 'Beautiful, isn't it, doctor? But after I have taken an injection it becomes exquisite.'

A few months after his apomorphine treatment in London, Burroughs wrote:

Tanger extends in several directions. You keep finding places you never saw before . . . Objects, sensations hit with the impact of hallucination. I now see with the child's eyes, the Lazarus eyes of return from the gray limbo of junk. But what I see is there. Others see it too.

– *Interzone*

Burroughs' literary resurrection had probably resulted from his withdrawal from the narcotic fog but after listening to my writer patient I began to wonder whether apomorphine itself might have been a contributory factor that allowed him to put the final touches to *Naked Lunch*.

Dr Dent put great store on the fact that apomorphine needed to be injected at regular 1–2 hour intervals around the clock for 7–10 days in order to be effective. He also stressed in his lectures that not a single one of his patients treated for anxiety rather than for alcoholism had ever become addicted to apomorphine.

The importance of following Dent's treatment protocol was further emphasised by Burroughs after his doctor's death:

It is essential to the success of the treatment to give a sufficient quantity of apomorphine over a sufficient period of time . . . With sublingual administration it is quite easy to control or eliminate nausea and the entire treatment can be carried out successfully without a single instance of vomiting. The concentration of apomorphine in the system must reach a certain level for the treatment to be successful. I have known doctors in America who gave two injections of apomorphine per day. This is quite worthless.
– *New Statesman*, 1966

The first patient I had seen with dopamine dysregulation had abused apomorphine by repeatedly injecting the drug whenever he began to feel he was switching off. We also saw several other patients who were overusing their 'rescue' shots. On the other hand the more severely disabled individuals who were being treated with the apomorphine pump rarely increased their dose and some voluntarily reduced it. I reasoned that repeated intermittent administration could subvert the dopamine system and lead to an increased wanting for apomorphine whereas delivery of the drug by infusion tonically stimulated the dopamine receptors and corrected the metabolic imbalance.

Neither Doctor Dent nor Burroughs were aware that apomorphine stimulated dopamine receptors. The important dopamine innervation of the limbic edge of the brain now known to be important for motivation and reward would not be discovered for another twenty years and the mapping of dopamine receptor reductions in drug addicts was a very recent finding. Dent's method was a rough approximation of the continuous stimulation of the dopamine receptors we had achieved with our apomorphine pumps.

As time passed, our radical suggestion of DOPA addiction in Parkinson's disease gained support, especially from experimental psychologists. Effective control of the motor symptoms in Parkinson's disease with L-DOPA or apomorphine could inadvertently lead to unwanted overdose effects on the relatively undamaged limbic and prefrontal dopamine pathways of the parkinsonian brain, culminating in undesirable cognitive and emotional changes.

The patients' narratives continued to spawn my research projects and led to fruitful collaborations with cognitive neuroscientists. Positron emission tomographic (PET) studies showed that L-DOPA had the capacity to induce procurement of more medication, irrespective of whether the effect of the drug was perceived to be pleasurable. The reward pathways had been sensitised resulting in an increased outpouring of dopamine. This in turn led to a heightened desire and an obligate requirement for more medication.

The seamstress told me that as long as she continued to organise her button collection she was able to prevent her DOPA 'switch offs'. Any attempt by her husband to stop her from punding was angrily resisted. The possibility that rewarding activities might offer new avenues of treatment for the 'on-off phenomenon' was completely unexplored. I took her anecdote as encouragement for future research.

Tim Lawrence, a young film stuntman with Parkinson's disease, had related on a BBC *Horizon* programme how he had inadvertently discovered that the Class A drug 'Ecstasy' (MDMA) had helped him to override his severe motor blocks. The TV footage showed him shedding his parkinsonian straitjacket and performing incredible dance floor backflips, swallow dives and somersaults. It seemed likely that Ecstasy was releasing large quantities of serotonin and this was having the effect of making his movements smoother and more fluid but I also wondered if the drug might be acting as a salient incentive for his dopamine reward system.

The chances of getting experiments involving 'Ecstasy' through the ethics committee and University College's Research and Development Department were small, so I settled on a test in which the patient volunteers would receive small financial gratuities for achieving card-sorting targets. The results revealed that patient volunteers with dopamine dysregulation and punding were more responsive to pecuniary inducement than matched patients with Parkinson's disease who had no addictive behaviour. One rewarded patient more than doubled his speed of sorting and switched spontaneously from 'off' to 'on' without the need for L-DOPA.

I had a hunch that this exaggerated feedback system for predicted rewards might stem from a more generalised effect of dopaminergic drugs like cocaine and amphetamine on the brain's motivational apparatus. The improvements seen with placebo medication in drug trials also probably occurred as a direct consequence of an increased surge of dopamine activity in the brain. The recognised healing powers of dance, exercise and music might also result from a fulfilling short-lived release of catecholamines.

After his successful withdrawal from junk, Burroughs had written to Dr Dent saying that he would be keen to collaborate on a book about narcotic addiction. His self-experimentation had provided me with insights into the cause of dependency and its treatment, and pointed the way towards a thesis. Not long after the publication of *Naked Lunch* in 1961, Burroughs was asked to deliver a paper at the 69th Annual Convention of the American Psychological Association in Manhattan on the differences between narcotics and psychedelic drugs. In his well-received talk he emphasised that exposure to drugs was always the first step on the road to addiction.

Burroughs knew all about the dissociation of liking from wanting, long before Berridge and Robinson's incentive salience theory was published in 1998. He also knew that junk laid down refractory narcotic memories by re-igniting processes involved in the normal ontogeny of reward circuits, and that effective treatment (permanent withdrawal) would require neuronal re-maturation.

He believed that all humans were hard-wired to be insatiable wanting machines. Sugar, laxatives and even shoplifting had the potential to become external objects of false satisfaction. Provided a novelty factor was introduced almost anything could be turned into a consumable. Corporations increased their stranglehold on the masses by alluring advertising. Junk was the ultimate merchandise and, in his paranoid but prescient world, a part of the global conspiracy.

To say it country simple, most folks enjoy junk. Having once experienced this pleasure, the human organism will tend to repeat it and repeat it and repeat it. The addict's illness is junk. Knock on any door. Whatever answers the door give it four and a half grain shots of God's Own Medicine every day for six months and the so called 'addict personality' is there.
– *New Statesman*, 1966

In further experiments carried out with the brain imagers at the Hammersmith Hospital, we were able to show that advertising (showing images of anti-Parkinson pills, food or sexually explicit pictures) reinforced dys-regulation in the DOPA addicts and suggested that be-havioural addictions like binge-eating and compulsive sexual disorder seen in some of the dopamine addicts could potentially increase drug wanting.

We next investigated the underlying cause for the 'overuse' of medication in the dysregulators. The beads task is a neuropsychological test that probes how much information an individual gathers before they make a decision. Research carried out with this test showed that both DOPA addicts and illicit drug users respond-ed far more rapidly and made more irrational choices than matched control groups, despite having intact working memories. This increased tendency to jump to conclusions without considering the consequences linked the Parkinson overusers to substance depend-ence and provided me with further evidence that the wanting of more and more L-DOPA was started and maintained by a destructive dopaminergic impulsivity rather than a loosening of the 'angels of restraint' in the inhibitory pre-frontal cortex.

Burroughs also anticipated the psychopharma-cological phenomenon of reinstatement whereby a mor-phine addict, abstinent from drugs for ten years, could become re-addicted after a single new exposure, where-as a newcomer to junk took at least six months to get hooked ('once a junky always a junky'). He also under-stood that the 'wanting system' became more active the less likely it was that an individual could obtain 'a hit'.

I openly recognised that Burroughs' raw data had informed the design of some of my experiments. It was all a matter of listening carefully to his wondrous flights of scientific fantasy. All he had ever wanted was to be part of the scientific debate but he had been excluded by a fellowship of personal interest. He had walked the talk but had been ignored.

By 2005 and before we had finished writing up all our research, dopamine had become a celebrity neurotransmitter, the 'sex drugs and rock and roll' hormone used by journalists along with brain imaging to give their clickable 'public awareness' news stories a scientific gloss. Anything that was desired and therefore potentially harmful was reported in the press as due to a rush of dopamine in the reward centres. Despite his mass of self-contradiction, Burroughs may well have had something important to say about this plethora of unscientific sloppy reportage and undue emphasis on sensationalist quantity over quality.

13

– The Bladerunner –

The bladerunner is a young man who supplies black market
medical supplies (including scalpel blades) for underground
medical practitioners in a dystopian futuristic Manhattan.
He was first conceived by Alan E. Nourse in his 1974 science
fiction novel *The Bladerunner* and has no direct connection
to Ridley Scott's film of the same name.

After his death in 1997, William Burroughs' insights
seemed to be even more connected to everything
and anything and his terrible predictions had come to
fruition. He was still a ghost in the soft machine but it
seemed that he had come to life. The past, present and
future all seemed to be happening at once.

The pharmaceutical industry was the largest
manufacturing industry in the world after the arms
business. Healthcare was a multi-billion pound
industry with ever increasing expenditure by tax-
payers that ultimately led to staggering profits for the
drug manufacturers. The pharmaceutical industry
was devoted to profit from illness and doctors were
a special interest group for disease preservation. The
government was a machine that fed off power. Profit-
driven medical science seemed determined to get the
whole world using pills.

I had now read all William Burroughs' published letters and paid close attention to many of his laser-sharp recordings. I had buried myself in *The Adding Machine*, *The Last Words*, *The Job*, *The Ticket that Exploded*, *Interzone*, *The Wild Boys*, *Cities of the Red Night* and *Nova Express* and learned a great deal from his *Paris Review* and *Playboy* interviews. Burroughs was suspicious of monopolies and authorities and the pyramid of dependencies created by post-war consumerism. Control would lead to greater control but could never be a means to a productive end. It was a virus that infested the human nervous system; only by eliminating fear could we wrest back autonomy.

I was still uncertain whether Burroughs had seen himself as a healer and a kind of voodoo scientist so I contacted James Grauerholz, who had first met him in 1974 and become his trusted companion, literary manager and adopted son. James had rescued Burroughs from a second treacherous descent into narcotic addiction during his residence in the Bowery. He wrote back on July 9 2014:

William had a complicated attitude toward doctors, and to unpack it requires one to distinguish doctors who were actually treating William, versus doctors whose published writings had come to William's attention – the Platonic Ideal of Doctorhood perhaps . . . For sure, he saw himself as some kind of doctor; he wanted to become a doctor – *und so weiter.*

In later correspondence James directed me to *Blade Runner: a movie*. This 1979 novella was Burroughs 'paste-in' companion to physician-writer Alan Nourse's science fiction novel. In the introduction Burroughs writes that the book is about the inflexibility and tunnel vision of vast service bureaucracies.

The story begins contemporaneously when overpopulation in America has led to ever-increasing government control over the citizen in the guise of a nanny state that dictates a citizen's terms of work, retirement benefits and medical care. Pressures are mounting for a National Health Act to impose a more equitable system of health care. After severe rioting in Manhattan and other American cities by the underclass, the National Health Act is passed, despite opposition from the drug corporations and private medical practitioners. Free healthcare finally becomes available to all citizens and residents of the United States of America. Nurses and doctors dance in the hospital corridors singing, 'The best things in life are free' and 'we belong to everybody'.

Within a generation of these reforms, average life expectancy has soared to 125, and is leading to a disturbing rise in the incidence of hereditary disorders, 'everybody would be diabetic or diabetes-prone by the late part of the next century'. New plagues of Alzheimer's and Parkinson's disease begin to emerge in the aged. A biomathematician predicts that the planet will soon be flooded with the worst samples of humanity with the lowest biological survival value. At the same time public health complacency is leading to the return of vanquished contagions like smallpox; the profligate use of antibiotics creates flesh-eating bugs.

By the end of the millennium, the government is becoming increasingly worried by reports of gangs of Naturist dogmatists demanding that all medicine be abolished. Senate rushes through an amendment to the National Health Bill stating that the 'unfit' (to be determined by a board of doctors and vaguely defined as a person over the age of five suffering from any form of hereditary disorder) are to be denied free health-care of any sort unless they agree to sterilisation. All doctors from now on will work only for the State and private practice will be banned.

By 2014, New York has become a world centre for underground medicine. Many roads are blocked with garbage and the potholes have been enlarged to serve as fishponds. Hydroponic guerrilla gardens flourish on rooftops, vacant lots and in basements. Treatments that could not be bought for any amount of money through official channels are now available in the back streets.

The shoestring entrepreneur, the innovator, the eccentric, the adventurer, long banished to limbo by the coalition of the big drug companies and the FDA, reappear.

More and more people are resisting the computerised regimentation of the State. Essential to this avant-garde network of experimental medicine are the blade runners who carry out the dangerous job of transferring medications and instruments from the research laboratories to the clandestine clinics.

Burroughs the mystagogue is describing the demise of totalitarian healthcare systems, predicting the appearance of apparently new viral diseases like AIDS and SARS, and anticipating virotherapy for cancer. Everything is fictional and at the same time everything seems prophetic.

When I had first read Ivan Illich in the seventies, his predictions of disaster had seemed too extreme. I was not wholly convinced that covetous doctors were causing more disease than they were curing and did not see why improved technology should automatically lead to less empathy or human care. I was also blasé about the potential harm done by wonder drugs. By the time I read *Blade Runner: a movie,* many of Illich's ideas had become mainstream. Something was now rotten in the state of medicine. Healthism had eaten up 17% of the US Gross Domestic Product. The worried well had been converted into patients by medical screening programmes and disease mongering (shyness and male baldness were considered ailments). Western healthcare systems – private or socialised – were new villains and doctors had been downgraded to menial technicians. Insurance companies were breaking down the art of accurate diagnosis in order to limit reimbursement. Ghost writers employed to write up commercially sponsored guideline documents in predatory open access journals were degrading the medical literature. The internet was the most potent cause of hypochondria that mankind had ever devised. Even the most sincere and reputable doctors now had vested interests.

Burroughs was imagining a new health model where people empower themselves to carry out their own experiments and provide their own alternative treatment. In these non-profit endeavours the people were prepared to challenge the authority of the State and take considerable risk. Some of the treatments available from the labs in the Lower City were highly dangerous and of unproven efficacy but this was viewed as an inevitable part of medical progress. People were making their own mind up about whether the risk was worth taking and carrying out their own investigation.

In a further letter, James reminded me that Burroughs had argued that the split between art and science needed to be healed urgently and that belief systems like chaos magic that came from territories outside scientific materialism should at least be explored. Science needed to be much more intuitive and magical and magic more factual and analytical. He was convinced human will could influence physical processes. He told Ted Morgan, his first biographer:

My viewpoint is the exact contrary of the scientific viewpoint.

I believe that if you run into somebody in the street it's for a reason. Among primitive people they say that if someone was bitten by a snake he was murdered. I believe that.

– *Literary Outlaw*

Burroughs opposed the exalted status given to medical scientists. They were imperfect individuals and their claim to an ultimate truth was false. Free will needed to be defended. In an interview with Allen Ginsberg published in *Journal for the Protection of All Beings* in 1961 he replied to a question about how technological society should be managed without controls:

Elimination of all natural sciences – If anybody ought to go to the extermination chambers, definitely scientists. Yes, I'm definitely anti-scientist because I feel that science represents a conspiracy to impose as the real and only universe, the universe of scientists themselves – they're reality-addicts, they've got to have things so real so they can get their hands on it.

The venal and self-serving Doc Benway used science as a strong form of control and a justification for his lack of humanity:

How in the fuck should I know? I'm a scientist. A pure scientist. Just get them outa here. I don't hafta look at them is all. They constitute an albatross.

– *Naked Lunch*

Doctor 'Fingers' Schafer began his presentation

at the International Conference of Technological Psychiatry with absolute conviction:

Gentlemen, the human nervous system can be reduced to a compact and abbreviated spinal column. The brain, front, middle and rear must follow the adenoid, the wisdom tooth, the appendix . . . I give you my Master Work: 'The Complete All American De-anxietized Man' . . .
– *Naked Lunch*

Burroughs was continuing to teach me things that had a direct bearing on modern medical practice. He made me entertain doubts about the dogmas of science and the preconceptions and received opinions that compromise objectivity. He reminded me to go on challenging authority and to try to break down my own ingrained outdated habits through mindfulness. *Blade Runner: a movie* was a warning that the National Health Service was under threat from Government appointed quangos and people who had no feel for what looking after sick people involves.

14

– Yagé Trip –

Although I knew that the few who had made land-mark contributions to the understanding of Parkinson's disease had done so while they were young, through an inevitable accident of time I now envisaged them as if they had always been venerable sages. James Parkinson, the patron saint of the shaking palsy, was the only notable exception, having been admitted to the inner sanctum at sixty-two years of age.

Parkinson was a radical and political pamphleteer, a palaeontologist of some distinction and a scientific conversationalist as well as being an apothecary. *An Essay on the Shaking Palsy* written in 1817, in which he describes six individuals he had observed during his travels through the Shoreditch streets, is a paragon of careful surveillance and accurate description. He hoped that his slim monograph would draw his medical colleagues' attention to a previously unclassified disorder, and stimulate the great anatomists of the day to locate the responsible lesion.

A wait of one hundred years then occurred before the cause for the slowness and stiffness was identified: a loss of melanin-containing nerve cells in the substantia nigra, a strip of nervous tissue in the midbrain. Then another fifty years passed before it was discovered that the nerve fibres projecting rostrally from the nigra to the corpus striatum ('striped body') contained dopamine. In 1990, lesions in the subthalamic nucleus of Luys in green monkeys provided evidence that excessive electrical activity in some regions of the basal ganglia circuitry occurred in Parkinson's disease and provided the rationale for deep brain stimulation with intracerebral electrodes.

Single-mindedness, dedication and a sprinkling of good fortune had allowed those responsible for these key breakthroughs to improvise their accumulated knowledge in resourceful new ways. Fortuitous events, seemingly unrelated to their work but dependent on their own particular interests, had played a part in their momentous discoveries.

In 1997, a gene responsible for parkinsonism was found in an extended Italian family – the alpha synu-clein mutation. This was saluted by the scientific press as the first identifiable cause of Parkinson's disease and despite the great rarity of the mutation it led to a sea change in the approach to research. Since then a great deal of enquiry has focused on the regulation of alpha synuclein in cells and its interaction with other mol-ecules. Alpha synuclein is a ubiquitous protein that is bound to membranes in nerve endings and is impor-tant for the trafficking of storage vesicles. Nerve cells communicate by a process that is part electrical and part chemical. The signal that passes along the nerve fibre is electrical but when it reaches the end of the axon, neurotransmitter packages stored in tiny envelopes called vesicles take over. If the highly regulated release of dopamine from these tiny pools is disrupted, electrical traces can no longer be transmitted to neighbouring nerve cells and the circuits go down. If alpha synuclein is the Rosetta Stone for Parkinson's disease then the cellular damage responsible for the symptoms of the illness must extend far beyond the substantia nigra and even beyond the brain.

Alpha synuclein misfolds and sticks together inside neurons, slowly choking up the motor highways and slowing the essential transport of cellular proteins. This causes the nerve fibres to die back, eventually causing nerve cell death. If the cascade of chemical reactions that triggers this abnormal protein clumping can be worked out, a new therapeutic era of vaccines and 'synuclein busters' might emerge.

The chastening reality, however, is that despite these scientific breakthroughs in our understanding and the investment of billions of pounds by the pharmaceutical industry, no treatment superior to L-DOPA has been developed. The last effective treatment to be marketed for Parkinson's disease in the United Kingdom is a L-DOPA gel (Duodopa) that has to be infused directly into the gut through a gastrostomy tube and costs the taxpayer a ludicrous £35,000 per patient per year.

Knowing of my interest in Burroughs, my research

team presented me with the mimeograph Apo-33 *Bulletin: A Medical Regulator; A Report on the Synthesis of the Apomorphine Formula* distributed by City Lights, San Francisco. On the front was a picture of the label from a box of the apomorphine hydrochloride pellets identical to the ones we had used in some of our early clinical trials.

Apo-33, written in crude type with rub-outs and sprinkled with barely legible printed handwriting, was Burroughs' prescription for society's ills. He now felt that his earlier account of apomorphine published in the *British Journal of Addiction* had been an edited cop out:

My attempt to attribute good will where it patently does not exist proved ill advised. I see no reason at this point to pull punches in the expectation of popularity.

The academic medical press was just another arrow in the quiver of the pharmaceutical establishment. It controlled information about addiction and apomorphine in the same way mainstream publishers stifled innovation and radical thought in creative writing. Guerilla writing in little magazines was Burroughs' best defence.

By the time Apo-33 had been published in 1965, he had realised that the medical industry was not going to share his optimistic view of apomorphine. He wrote that the American Narcotics Department and

Public Health Service were errand boys for the White Goddess and were paid in White Junk. Medical science was determined to reduce the whole of mankind to the helplessness of addicts. A drug-free, phobia less society was inconceivable; the political stakes were too high.

He wrote that apomorphine, 'like a good policeman did its work and left no trace'. It steadied the system and regulated the body in the same way cut-up writing regulated the power of the word. It was through reading *Apo-33* that I first appreciated Burroughs' views of the controlling power of language. It made me think about how important the right word was at the right time in medical practice, but also how often a healing silence had come to my aid in response to anguish and despair.

By 2010, the feelings of alienation I had experienced as a final year medical student had returned and were slowly turning me into a belated but committed freedom fighter. I could now see much more clearly where things were going wrong. Many of my colleagues shared similar opinions and we celebrated our occasional small victories against the Clinical Directorate with childish pleasure. The National Health Service regarded neurology as an expensive, largely talking speciality with woolly outcomes and there was never enough funding. Performance was now judged by waiting times, not quality of care or innovation. Professionalism was being replaced by brainless accountability reflected in meaningless league tables. After the serial murders committed by Doctor Harold Shipman had been uncovered, no practitioners were to be trusted; after the Alder Hey Hospital organ scandal all pathologists were suspect. Burroughs' bête noires from *Apo-33* had been joined by some new and less publicised tyrannies.

In the pretence to be more scientific, only the very latest and most immediate data was now considered trustworthy. Painstaking, clinical, pharmacological observation in small numbers of patients was disparaged as 'eminence based medicine.' New was better than old, more was superior to little, complex always trumped simple, and early detection of disease was essential – such truisms reflected the prevailing zeitgeist.

A culture that encouraged freedom, intellectual diversity, flexibility, and originality, had been very much in evidence when I first began my research at University College Hospital. Scientific collaboration then was based on equality and contribution, not authoritative commands delivered from on high. In 1990, I had obtained permission from the UCH Research and Ethics Committee, the Metropolitan Police and the Home Office to carry out a trial of marijuana cigarettes in Parkinson's disease. The trial had been suggested by one of my patients who had observed that when she smoked cannabis her tremor disappeared for several hours. The volunteers puffed 'joints' on Jack Hambro Ward at the Middlesex Hospital while we recorded the drug's effect on their tremor and slowness. The results of our trial were negative but the role of cannabinoids in the treatment of neurological disease later became an area of intense research interest. Such a proof of principle study would now be deemed bad research and not allowed even though it had revived interest in a forgotten treatment.

Lack of trust and a culture of patient complaining encouraged by government and consumer organisations were further new serious roadblocks. Younger colleagues who were keen to do research were buckling under the sheer volume of inflexible rules, auditing and clinical guidelines. The regulations governing who paid for what in research in the National Health Service were a complex jumble, quite beyond the comprehension of most mortals. The Data Protection Act was another obstruction. After ethical approval, every study involving data from National Health Service records required an application to the Patient Information Advisory Group. If approval was granted the project then had to be reviewed annually to ensure the investigators were moving towards informed consent or anonymisation. Before 1998 I had tried to answer a few of the numerous clinical uncertainties that still existed in everyday neurological practice through 'reviews of case notes' at the National Hospital, seldom with permission from the patients but without a single complaint. This was now out of the question without going through months of cumbersome officialdom.

Policing of research had become extraordinarily bureaucratic, expensive and confusing. Although ethics committees provided necessary protection against research subjects being harmed, the time researchers now had to spend to obtain approval even for minor amendments to their protocol was lengthy. University Research and Development departments, however well intentioned, had bogged down researchers with their unnecessary bean counting and legalistic red tape. They were a cancerous growth eating away at novelty. The big lie was that they were necessary to protect society from maverick physicians conducting poor research. The 'little men' like Patrick Steptoe (in vitro fertilisation pioneer) and John Charnley (the man who invented hip replacement) had been extinguished because they did not have the resources or desire to comply with this judgemental administration. A body that had been set up to support and assist researchers had worked against many of them. Blue sky innovation by individuals rather than corporations was stifled whereas derivative research that fitted a standard and recognised format was condoned. Compliance with the rules was now prohibitively expensive except for industry, meaning that the research agenda would be inevitably shaped by profit. The emphasis was on process and political correctness, not ethics or good science. What was even worse was the fact that these bodies within universities were colluding with funders, journals and science leaders to cover up malpractice.

In some situations over-regulation had led to serious bias with wrong conclusions being drawn. For example if the individual's right to opt out is extended too far then the collected data will come from a biased sample because those patients who agree to their data being used may be very different from those who don't.

Lobbying scientists, media professors and self-satisfied cliques of super-specialists who met periodically to pat themselves on the back and forecast the future were new forces purporting to represent science. Many of these people seemed to believe that research papers were literary products and science was a continuation of politics by another means. Others had grossly over optimistic expectations of the clinical benefits of basic biological research. Medical journals and researchers now counted any media coverage as a good thing and would overextend their results in press releases to sell it. It seemed to me that academic medicine had been hijacked by basic science and was not fit for purpose.

Everything was now constrained, governed and directed by rules, nothing was possible. Exploitation, abuse and an oppressive bumbledom had not been included in my job plan but I felt acutely aware of all three now. I gave up on one academic clinical pharmacological study after a battle of more than a year, in which despite obtaining funding, ethical approval and free samples of the already licensed drug from the manufacturer, the Hospital Trust where I had worked for thirty years refused to accept indemnity. Some of the desperate patients whom I had told about the proposed study were disappointed when I informed them that unfortunately the trial was not to go ahead. Some offered to sign a consent form that would divorce the hospital from any indemnity for their well-being and safety. In my experience most patients understand that better clinical care depends on research. Many comment that in course of a trial they receive better follow-up, enjoy more time with the doctor, and are given better information about their illness. In a trial I had conducted many years ago, before the routine availability of brain scans, a research volunteer who was acting as a control was found to have a large 'silent' tumour, which if it had not been picked up and operated on may well have left him with serious neurological deficit.

When I sought advice from The Medical Defence Union, the body I paid to provide me with legal support should my competence be questioned, I was advised that it would be unwise to proceed because it would be difficult to defend me if one of the consented patients went back on their word and sued. In other words the patient's word was not worth the paper it was written on. In the end, my longstanding deep-seated fear of authority prevented me from pressing ahead. The officials and the apparatchiks had won the day while the ever longer delays in sanctioning fresh research were costing lives.

Of greater concern than the lack of new treatments in Parkinson's disease was the fact that some of the useful, cheap drugs that had been approved in the NICE National Guidelines for Parkinson's disease, like amantidine, benzhexol and Sinemet, kept inexplicably disappearing from pharmacies all over the country, leaving patients and their doctors to manage potentially life-threatening, acute, unsupervised drug-withdrawals. The Government took no responsibility for guaranteeing drug supplies or curbing market forces, leading to a system that allowed retail warehouses to sell their stocks for more money to other European countries. Once a drug had become cheap and unprofitable, it was at risk of abandonment even when it was the best available remedy. In keeping with the lamentable reporting of important health issues in the British press, this scandal received scant and low-key coverage.

In 1776, James Parkinson had been admitted as a pupil to my alma mater. As my career had advanced, his optimism expressed in *An Essay on the Shaking Palsy* had often spurred me on:

On the contrary, there appears to be sufficient reason for hoping that some remedial process may ere long be discovered, by which, at least the progress of the disease may be stopped.

I badly wanted to make up for lost time, overcome the challenges and make Parkinson's prediction come true. Many important and tractable basic clinical questions had remained ignored and unanswered, to the disappointment of my patients. The solution was clear. I needed to forge alliance with groups representing patients with Parkinson's disease in order to break free.

In 1995, at a time when my research group had been investigating the therapeutic potential of a new reversible type A monoamine oxidase inhibitor called moclobemide, I had alighted upon a review article by Juan Sánchez-Ramos from the University of Miami. He described a fascinating bygone chapter in the history of neurological therapeutics that gave me hope that Burroughs had been right and that yagé, despite its inherent dangers, might yet be 'the final fix'.

Louis Lewin, the Berlin pharmacologist who had isolated harmine (banisterine) from the B. caapi stems, had described feelings of re-invigoration and faster reactions after self-experimentation. He had then administered the drug to an obese patient in the Neuekolin Hospital who described immediate lightness of her limbs and an improved speed of walking. Encouraged by the alkaloid's effects on movement he suggested that banisterine might offer hope for sufferers with postencephalitic Parkinson's syndrome (the sleepy sickness survivors). As he was approaching retirement, he recommended that two younger colleagues, Beringer and Willmans, should conduct the first trials in Heidelberg.

Beringer, who had published papers on mescaline-induced visions and their relevance to schizophrenia, administered 100 mg of harmine to a volunteer colleague and noted 'an uncontrollable tremor in the arms and legs, similar to what we see in parkinsonian patients'. Despite this setback he proceeded to treat fifteen postencephalitic patients and captured striking improvements in their mobility if not their tremor on a series of cinematographic recordings. One of the patients who had been incapacitated by stiffness and had a spasm of the jaw told him, 'Doctor, I am healthy again'. Benefit from harmine was seen after about thirty minutes and in some cases lasted for many hours.

Within a year of Beringer's published findings in 1928, the Merck Company marketed harmine for the treatment of parkinsonism and made it available to doctors in capsules, suppository and injectable form. Nineteen pages of the *Merck Jahrbuch* were devoted to its potential as a neurotropic agent and the company's literature particularly recommended it for younger patients with Parkinson's disease who had no tremor. Beringer warned his medical colleagues of unrealistic expectations and cautioned that the 'exaggerated and extravagant reports in the newspapers' were 'arousing hopes in the ill that could not be fulfilled'. He drew attention to the variability and unpredictability of harmine's effect. While some patients had spectacularly improved, others had no benefit and in one or two, tremor had worsened. In 1930, a German physician named Halpern took a dose of 40 mg by mouth and wrote:

The impression was felt as if consciousness was packed in ether. When lying on a sofa, the light-headedness increased to a feeling of floating and the weight of the body was subjectively less. These clinical observations should be compared to the state of levitation frequently reported to occur with the crude drug ayahuasca or caapi . . . With higher doses excitation was increased even in an aggressive way . . . the author who is normally not belligerent started a fight with a man in the street where he was the one who attacked even though according to the circumstances the prospect for the attacker was unfavourable.

In the 1 March 1929 edition of the periodical *Charon-nothefte; der kompass,* harmine was heralded as a magic formula and its use spread rapidly throughout continental Western Europe. But by 1932 the high hopes for the drug had all but gone and harmine experienced a fall from grace almost as precipitous as had been its sensational uptake. It still had a few advocates and in 1945 Dr Morell asked Ludwig Stumpfegger to treat Adolf Hitler's parkinsonism with Merck's harmine.

Many of the potions that were used to treat Parkinson's disease in the nineteenth and first half of the twentieth century such as calabar beans, Raeff's Bulgarian belladonna concoction, henbane, monkey glands, iron carbonate, and parathyroid extract had rightly been discarded. Only synthetic drugs like trihexiphenidyl (Artane) and orphenadrine (Disipal), whose introduction had hastened the demise of harmine survived and remain useful for the control of rigidity, trembling and spasms. Harmine had never been marketed for depression but the improvements we had seen with moclobemide, the new type A monoamine oxidase inhibitor, in both depression and motor handicap in Parkinson's disease, kept the flame alive. I had also learned from this paper that yagé was used as a religious sacrament by two state-approved churches in Brazil (União do Vegetal and Santo Daime).

I next came across another paper in a scarcely-read journal by Dr Marcos Serrano Dueñas, a neurologist working in Quito and Dr Sánchez-Ramos, the author of the banisterine review paper. They had carried out a trial in which thirty previously untreated patients with Parkinson's disease had been randomised to receive either 200 ml of *Banisteriopsis caapi* extract or 200 ml of an equally bitter-tasting placebo drink. Highly significant improvements in speed of movement and reductions in stiffness had been seen in the active treatment arm, with feelings of sickness and diarrhoea as the only reported adverse effects. In common with Beringer's earlier results a worsening of tremor occurred in one or two cases. The dosage the patients received was equivalent to the brew Schultes' Desana Indian guide had provided Burroughs with and which he had found rather disappointing as a hallucinogen. No researchers or phytopharmaceutical companies pursued these findings and the article had plummeted into the annals of neglected medical literature. The only interest in the paper had come from the medical department of the União do Vegetal. Sanchez-Ramos was invited to present his results at their scientific meeting held in 1992 at the Hotel Gloria in Rio de Janeiro, where cultural and scientific ideas were exchanged relating to caapi as a promoter of health, serenity and wellbeing and its potential as a treatment for nervous ailments.

The apomorphine saga had taught me that the excavation and re-investigation of remedies consigned to oblivion was an alternative to the 'bench to bedside' idyll of academic medicine. Colleagues I spoke to who were employed in the pharmaceutical industry informed me that there were hundreds of unremembered molecules of potential interest sitting on dusty shelves waiting for a plug. They also told me there were virtually no company-sponsored botanists going into the forests as Spruce and Schultes had done.

I wanted to believe that these more striking results with the stems of the natural vine compared with Merck's harmine were due to an 'entourage effect' in which whole plant extracts could produce better results than the purified alkaloid.

At my request, Serrano-Dueñas posted several

dried B. caapi stems and together with Peter Houghton and Peter Jenner at King's College London we went on to demonstrate that both harmine and harmaline, identified in the plant material, could release dopamine as well as prevent the neurotransmitter's breakdown by type A monoamine oxidase inhibition.

By 2010, government funding had dwindled and the big pharmaceutical companies had all but baled out from drug development in Parkinson's disease. The flow of new drugs had reduced to a trickle and the patients' hopes for a fast cure now lay largely in the hands of venture capitalists, wealthy private benefactors and charitable foundations. Any treatment that came through had a new hurdle to overcome which had nothing to do with science. Payers employed by the Department of Health and private insurance companies were now a very important consideration in what had become a 3.5 billion dollar game.

Drug company sponsored trials had become rewarding for NHS Trust hospitals but they were colossal and impersonal. Data collection from the patient volunteers involved a mechanical, tedious process of box-ticking dictated by the European Medicines Agency and the FDA rather than scientific rationale or even common sense. The Trust often delegated this time-consuming chore involving kilograms of paper to research nurses whose salaries were funded partly by the pharmaceutical company and who did not mind if their name was not included on the eventual publication. Clinical trials now took three times longer than in 1975 and were infinitely more expensive to conduct. Less than one in ten drugs in development made it all the way to the clinic. The heroic era of neuropharmacological research had long vanished and self-experimentation was denigrated for its danger and lack of objectivity. Burroughs' dream that molecules more potent and less toxic than yagé could be synthesised and find wider medical application had been ignored. Parkinson's disease research went round in circles with no beginnings and no end. Treatments came and went according to fashion.

—

In my sixty-sixth year I prepared myself for a new journey of radical empiricism. Although I had failed in my adolescent desire to follow in the footsteps of Richard Spruce, I had made many contacts with Brazilian neurologists and a meeting of the Brazilian Academy of Neurology to which I was invited in Belém in 2013 finally provided the excuse I had been waiting for. Hallucinogenic molecules could open up frightening new vistas of exploration and if Burroughs was right, my trip to the Amazon would lead me to unimagined cures. I wanted to see whether yagé could infuse my monochromatic research canvas and open up vivid new scientific perspectives.

I arrive by boat at Tabatinga and climb up the jetty looking for a ride to Colombia. Surrounded on all sides by motorcycles, I bump across the coca frontiers on a tuk tuk past the Hotel Anaconda and the deafening screech of the roosting parakeets in Parque Santander. At Kilometros Seis we turn off Via Leticia and pass a barrier guarded by a languorous guard before entering the shadowy *aldeia* of the tree spirits.

Dona Angélica Floréz is a slight, white-haired storyteller with an interest in the unpredictable and a clairvoyant gift. She shares her name with a celestial tree with starburst flowers that is used to promote healing and remove curses. She was born north of the Putumayo in La Chorrera, a municipality notorious during the rubber boom for some of Casa Arana's worst atrocities. Her family had moved to Leticia at the time of the hostilities between Colombia and Peru in 1932. Her abode is sparsely furnished with a firewood hearth and with a few fading magazine cuttings on the wall. At the back of the house, a door leads out to a patio where a liana with winged fruits coils up a wall and angel's trumpet flowers open in anticipation of the early evening moths. Dona Angélica's Indian eyes are like dark mysterious pools. I follow her through the small garden into a dark wooden cabin.

She sits on the stone floor and puts on a white *Arara* headdress and beaded necklace. In front of her on a low circular table are four dirty plastic bottles, a heap of fresh leaves and some pieces of vine. I drink the sour dark liquid from a calabash. An intense nausea coming straight from the brain is my first reaction to the brew. The room is silent and soon the candle is extinguished. In the darkness the croak of the yellow dart frog, the sound of children playing in the street outside and the roar of a plane heading for Tabatinga, all seem abnormally penetrating. I feel cold and pensive. Angélica begins to intone in her quivering, sibilant voice. I close my eyes, hunch forward and begin to see preternatural apparitions just beneath my eyelids, a gallimaufry of ever changing faces, an unrecognizable metropolis and the buttresses of Gormenghast. As I travel through inner space, motion sickness comes in stomach-churning gusts. I feel near death. Angélica continues to calm me with her haunting singing. After a long time a *curandero* called Juan anoints my face and hands with camphor, brushes me with a knotted sprig of leaves and invokes the healing spirits of the trees and the waters.

I am under the influence of a strong force carrying me higher and faster through space. I begin to imagine scenes that have not yet happened and which I cannot understand. A soft whistling incantation breaks the silence. Yellow and green iridescent zigzag spectra and indigo and argent helices are under my eyes, ultramarine charges come out of my arms. Jungles glide past and I see vast rivers of land accelerating past locked shorelines. Without opening my eyes I can see a tableau of the sad history of Iquitos, and in my sunlit Cabinet of Curiosity, large numbers of morphos with seven-inch wingspans and green-blue shimmering wings arrive to mate. Their iridescence and wobbling flight is a symbol of the perfection of the forest. Their burnished, metallic gloss creates the appearance of a perfect mosaic on the back of my hand. Time and causality seem abhorrent. Yagé confirms my belief that I am just an element linked inextricably to a whole and that I can never stand apart. The flashes of beauty intensify as I stagger from the lodge. Outside on the leaden street I see gleaming fireflies among the phantom moths. Phosphenes, coiled floating chains and *aerolitos* flash above me. Images unwind from the windmills of my mind. The journey back to the hotel is a spellbinding trip in another dimension with throbbing stars and lime disco lights. I am seeing things from a special angle. The black trees convey a divine unspoken message from the land.

As I lurch from the bedroom to the bathroom my body seems to be creating lurid serpentine tints that zip across the wall like electric storms. I feel invisible raindrops on my arms as I am propelled on a beautiful aquamarine tide. In the gleaming of day I now know that rational consciousness is parted by the thinnest of films from illusion and dream. Seeing things that are not there can occur in the blind, the bereaved and even in waking dreams. The innate knowledge of the Amazon Indian assisted by the ritual use of sacred plants has given me second sight. I understand for

the first time how during hurricanes, chairbound victims of Parkinson's disease can magically override the
poltergeist and escape to safety. The plant teachers,
through their 'doctoritos' (little doctors) had shifted
my understanding of reality. I now could see into my
own mind.

15

– Altamirage –

E ncountering William Burroughs when I was a student had been a fortunate accident that had almost culminated in me rejecting medicine for a life of vagabondage. He was the Pied Piper of Hamelin hungry for revenge against all those doctors who had reduced the sanctity of the consultation to a transaction and who had chosen to ignore the importance of silent waiting. He was the ugly, self-indulgent spirit who haunted my dreams with his lurid descriptions of hanging. His gallows humour had helped me break through my own hang-ups and recognise evil.

Goodness had finally pulled me back from a chasm of disappointment. I saw love and kindness in operation every day in the hospital. I enjoyed attending the neurologically sick and the intellectual challenge of medicine. Through stories transmitted from one generation of physicians to the next, neurology had come alive. I considered myself very fortunate to have been given the chance to be a doctor even though I continued to doubt the value and wisdom of what I did on a daily basis. The medical profession had saved me and kept the wolf from the door.

One patient with Parkinson's disease told me that

in some ways the illness had been a blessing. It had allowed him to become more contemplative, liberated him from the rat race and saved him from drink. Another told me that instead of waiting for something to strike her down, she knew exactly what she was up against.

But on those occasional days when attending the neurologically ill was not enough to fill my heart and mind, Burroughs' non-linear presence sustained me. He was now a symbol of unlimited scientific possibility, the archangel of abundance who guided me beyond the far horizon and encouraged my wistfulness:

This is the space age and we are here to go. However, the space programme has been restricted so far to a mediocre elite who at great expense have gone to the moon in an aqualung. Now they are not really looking for space they are looking for more time like the lungfish and the walking catfish they were not really looking for new dimensions different from water they were looking for more water. But some of them found that they had taken an irretrievable forward step and for better or worse left their gills to their makers. And as we leave the aqualung of time we may step into an epic comparable to the days when the early mariners set out to explore an unknown world.

– Nova Convention, 30 November–2 December 1978, New York City

My peregrination to the Amazon had convinced me that most pharmaceutical companies were either uninterested in Parkinson's disease or on the wrong track. Many chief executive officers in Pharma now had a background in business management or international law and had no feel for how research operated. Most proclaimed that science was primarily about creating wealth.

Increases in the cost of new drugs, aggressive advertising directly to consumers and suppression of negative trial data were cynical ploys now used by the pharmaceutical companies to maximise profit for shareholders. Sharks in suits and good 'company players' flourished in disjointed multinational outfits and were rewarded with promotion or pay-offs for bad decision-making and failure. The dwindling number of smaller companies who still tried to foster individual freedom and inspiration in their beleaguered medical departments were constantly strapped for cash and in danger of take-over. 'Benchmarking' had resulted in the Pharma giants ignoring their particular areas of expertise, and becoming more and more like each other.

The complex, lengthy and ever more expensive process of bringing a drug to market had led to a current attrition rate of more than 90%, even when a compound had entered clinical development. An institutional lack of imagination and cowardice had resulted in the premature curtailment of the development of many promising molecules.

The paradox of the modern clinical trial was that

even if it was the best way to assess whether a new intervention worked, it was the worst way to assess who would benefit from it. Statistically significant results sufficient to obtain a product licence frequently translated to negligible advantage for the individual. I knew instinctively that multicentre trials with so many exclusion criteria, even if considered Level 1 evidence with Grade A recommendations, would only ever form a small part of my bedside clinical decision-making. Best medical treatment depended not only on the quality of the proof but the context in which it was applied and required expert judgement rather than unemotional conformity. The patient should always come first.

Botany, *Sergeant Pepper's Lonely Hearts Club Band* and the great Portuguese navigators had informed all my modest medical discoveries. Research was a series of loops that sometimes doubled back before it moved forward. My experience had taught me that the art of the soluble was constructed from a series of zigzags, joined by the most fragile of links. My best ideas had flickered in from the margins of consciousness and had taken root on the frontiers between bewilderment and understanding. I saw science as a tempest of thought threads that collided and interacted continually. The book of Nature had remained open before me revealing a chaotic resonating world where nothing was impossible.

After my trip to the Amazon I had managed to dismantle some restrictive frames of reference, and in the space that opened up I determined to re-investigate

Banisteriopsis caapi (yagé) as a medicine. I had been chasing my tail, stuck in a rut and missing the way forward. I was now determined to force Nature to unveil herself in response to my questions.

With colleagues at Kings College, we began work to examine whether B.caapi could reverse the signs of Parkinson's disease in MPTP treated marmosets. MPTP was the protoxin taken by the six Californian drug addicts in 1982 that had caused them to seize up and which now was considered to be the best, if imperfect, animal model of the shaking palsy. At the same time I also began to plan a clinical trial with neurologists at the Federal University of Rio de Janeiro in collaboration with a botanist at the Jardim Botanico who would provide the vine and its certificate of authenticity. We hoped to recruit some patient volunteers for the trial from members of the União do Vegetal Church who already imbibed the vine as part of the holy sacrament.

Perhaps yagé would one day take its place alongside the other treatments for Parkinson's disease, and the stunning magnificence of its phosphenes would increase inner space exploration. It might also aid the human spirit to comprehend its true transcendent nature and eliminate all fear. I felt sure, after my own experience, that there was something in it.

At the same time as I started this new research with the vine of the soul, I also started to follow up on my aporphine research that had also been driven by Burroughs' writing. I contacted John Neumeyer, whose work I had admired ever since I started to use apomorphine but whom I had never had the chance to meet. John was a medicinal chemist working at Harvard whose family had been forced to leave Nazi Germany during World War II. He had done much of his secondary education in Manchester before his family immigrated to America. John was not a fraudster and had not been driven during his long distinguished scientific career by fame or greed. He wrote back to me immediately:

Dear Professor Lees,

Thank you for your email and for contacting me regarding Apomorphine. We too have found little interest from the pharma industry in funding any of this research but in the last 10 years a chemist friend with deep pockets and suffering from Parkinson's disease has generously funded our research program here at McLean Hospital. I would be delighted to collaborate with you in your endeavour to develop orally active analogs of apomorphine for clinical investigation. Our problem has been to find interested pharmacologist and clinicians to further such studies.

I look forward to your further correspondence.

Sincerely,

John L. Neumeyer

P.S. Reading Naked Lunch by William Burroughs in 1965 was the stimulus for me to focus on APO and its pharmacology.

I now had a serious partner and kindred spirit who had also responded to Burroughs lament:

Pharmaceutical researchers are told what research to pursue by vested interest, which gives orders to the American Narcotics Department. Billions for variations on the Benzedrine formula, for tranquilizers of dubious value, not ten cents for a drug that has unlimited potentials not only in treating addiction but in handling the whole problem of anxiety.

– *The Job*

John synthesised a batch of an aporphine called R (-) 11-Hydroxy-N-n-propylnoraporphine which he believed, based on its conformational structure, would have strong dopamine-stimulating effects. I also had a benefactor with Parkinson's disease who was prepared to give us both a chance. With this philanthropic financial assistance we were able to join forces with colleagues at Kings College and demonstrate that John's molecule fulfilled all Burroughs' criteria. It was long-acting, powerful and most importantly, worked when given by mouth.

After the marmoset experiments finished and the manuscript had been sent for publication, John sent me a gift of *VINE of the SOUL, Medicine Men, their Plants and Rituals in the Colombian Amazonia* that his former friend and colleague Dick Schultes had signed.

Our paper was accepted for publication after I had been able to reassure the editor that a pharmaceutical company was seriously interested in gambling on our findings. Thirty million pounds would be needed to take the molecule from the monkey laboratory through to multicentre trials in patients. Those risk-taking deprenil days, where informative research could be done on a shoestring, seemed like a distant faraway world.

Burroughs had become an unlikely prognosticator and a trusted oracle. He reminded me to be open minded and non-judgemental and run with what life

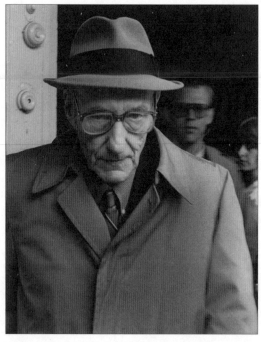

Burroughs in the doorway of Atticus Bookshop, Liverpool,
5 October 1982

threw my way. He emphasised I should never miss a chance. He looked at the literature in a slanted and unusual way. He showed me that dead ends were part of scientific research and that I should never rule anything out. He had taught me that I had the capacity to work miracles but at the same time I needed to be sceptical. He taught me that egotism and single-mindedness were prerequisites for research and that science had always followed Jesus not Marx. He encouraged me to get away from concrete thinking, float in outer space and to run alongside a beam of light. He also reminded me that clinical investigation should not be limited to institutions and that scientists must find new ways to regain the power to explore. He studied things that mattered to all mankind and had tried to work out why most human beings behaved like idiots. He dissected intelligence with a naturalist's stance and carried out a meticulous examination of everything he turned his attention to. He added a strange grace to my research that helped me to fly crookedly in my curiosity for cures.

He was not interested in relieving human suffering, but the fusion of his ideas with my own scientific meanderings had allowed me to see things in a completely different light. He realised that science was blinding medicine and healthcare was ripping off its customers. I shared his view that the blunt rationalism of society's control mechanisms was arresting human development and had started to cause self-harm and destruction of the environment. As the world's rainforests came down and human greed made more and more animals extinct, the ability to imagine and mythologise was in danger of disappearing and dying too. Burroughs feared our dreams were being cut off at source.

John and I were swimming against the tide of scientific fashion and following Burroughs' apomorphine mantra. We were being blown by a strong wind through a crimson sky, upwards to the star cities in the Milky Way. Immersed in cloud we saw new symmetries amid the changing shapes of molecules. We were prepared to leave behind everything we had ever known. Time was our resource but it was running short. We still had hopes of blazing a trail among the Pleiades.

– Acknowledgements –

I never met William Burroughs but he helped me realise I was not unreal or alone in this vast immensity of space and time. Several members of the 'Burroughs Establishment', an oxymoron if ever there was one, gave my literary experiment the nudge it needed to reach completion. Their munificence and openness stemmed from their viewpoint rather than any surprise and pleasure that a neurologist might be interested in their specialist subject.

James Grauerholz has become my 'epistolary audience' and sage. We have exchanged reams of light hearted but informative correspondence about 'the madman'. He has shared with me some of his own unpublished writing and an annotated copy of an article by Peter Swales entitled *Burroughs in the Bewilderness, The Haunted Mind and Psychoanalyses of William S. Burroughs* that has never been published. He has also played a crucial role in helping me break through my hang-ups. Oliver Harris encouraged me to look at Burroughs' work from a scientific viewpoint and invited me to join a group of deadbeats (The European Beat Studies Network) whose imagination has no limits. Isabelle Aubert-Baudron, curator of Interzone, a liberated network of collective intelligence for Burroughs readers, advised me to confront the unknown.

Bill Morgan helped me particularly with the links between Burroughs and the Baker Street sleuth and Mike Jay, that rare animal, the independent scholar, gave me shrewd advice based on his encyclopaedic knowledge of the cultural history of medicine and science. Jim Pennington, Editor and Investigator at Aloes Books, provided invaluable arcane snippets from the sixties that inform some of the key illustrations.

Juana Luisa Pulin, my wife, who has had more than her fill of listening to Burroughs' instantly recognisable drawl, is my eternal muse. Maurice Earls, editor of the *Dublin Review of Books*, who published my essay 'Hanging around with the Molecules' in 2014 and Robert McCrum, who took up the story in the *Observer*, both merit my gratitude. I also wish to thank Tom Kremer, the founder of Notting Hill Editions, for taking a risk on a most implausible association.

Warwick Sweeney provided personal details about his grandfather Dr John Dent and encouraged me with his spirited epistles. He also allowed me to publish correspondence between Dent and Burroughs. Mark Seaward, lichenologist and botanical historian, tracked down the recherché texts that conclusively linked Burroughs to the unravelling of the mysteries of yagé. Geoff Ward, Jill McArdle and Tom Flemons supplied essential detail of the one and only visit William Burroughs made to Liverpool.

Most editors of medical scientific books do little more than badger and harry the authors to deliver their chapters by deadline day. They rarely make suggestions as to how the content can be improved. In striking contrast and to my great relief, Kim Kremer, my editor, went through my manuscript rigorously and sensitively on three separate occasions and after each round of suggestions my readers were benefited.

My teachers and all the inspiring people with Parkinson's disease I have had the honour to treat may be surprised by this story but I hope they will not feel betrayed. Without them there is no mystery.

Much of *Mentored by a Madman: The William Burroughs Experiment* was written in the contrasting but equally stimulating surroundings of the Caffé Paradiso on Store Street and the London Library in St James's Square but the tale was conceived in Liverpool at Kerouacs on Smithdown Road.

– Select Bibliography
of Works by William Burroughs –

Naked Lunch: The Restored Text (2015)
Junky: The Definitive Text of 'Junk' (2008)
The Yage Letters Redux (2008)
The Letters of William S. Burroughs, Volume 1 1945–1959
    (1993)
Rub Out the Words: Letters 1959–1974 (2013)
Last Words: The Final Journals (2001)
Burroughs Live: The Collected Interviews of William S.
    Burroughs, 1960–1997 (2002)
The Job Interviews with William S Burroughs (2008)
The Adding Machine (2013)
Blade Runner: a movie (2010)
Ghost of Chance (2002)
Apo-33 Health Bulletin: A Metabolic Regulator (1968)

Notting Hill Editions is devoted to the best in essay writing. Our authors, living and dead, cover a broad range of non-fiction, but all display the virtues of brevity, soul and wit.

Our commitment to reinvigorating the essay as a literary form extends to our website, where we host the wonderful Essay Library, a home for the world's most important and enjoyable essays, including the facility to search, save your favourites and add your comments and suggestions.

To discover more, please visit
www.nottinghilleditions.com

Other titles from Notting Hill Editions*

You and Me: The Neuroscience of Identity
by Susan Greenfield

What is it that makes you distinct from me? *You and Me*
considers the concept of identity from the perspective of a
neuroscientist. Greenfield takes us on a biological interpretation
of this most elusive of concepts.

'Greenfield is a lucid and thorough communicator'
– *The Independent*

My Katherine Mansfield Project
by Kirsty Gunn

In this lyrical essay, Gunn explores the idea of home and
belonging – and of the profound influence of Mansfield's work
on her own creative journey.

'I began reading it and could not put it down . . . It really lives,
all of it.' – John Carey

Pilgrims of the Air
by John Wilson Foster

The story of the rapid and brutal extinction of the Passenger
Pigeon, once so abundant that they 'blotted out the sky'.
It is also an evocative story of wild America – the ruthless
exploitation of its 'commodities', and a morality tale for our
times.

'Every page of this book is lit with a sense of wonder.'
– Michael Longley

Confessions of a Heretic
by Roger Scruton

A collection of hard-hitting essays by the influential social
commentator, Roger Scruton. Scruton challenges popular
opinion on key aspects of our culture and seeks to answer the
most pressing problems of our age.

Attention! A (short) history
by Joshua Cohen

A dazzling meditation on the philosophical, scientific and historical roots of attention, an attempt to pin down this elusive state of being.

'*Attention!* will allow you to smile, argue, agree, refute or just go along for an engaging ride.' – Jenni Diski, *Guardian*

CLASSIC COLLECTION

The Classic Collection brings together the finest essayists of the past, introduced by contemporary writers.

Beautiful and Impossible Things
– Selected Essays of Oscar Wilde
Introduced by Gyles Brandreth

Words of Fire – Selected Essays of Ahad Ha'am
Introduced by Brian Klug

Essays on the Self – Selected Essays of Virginia Woolf
Introduced by Joanna Kavenna

All That is Worth Remembering
– Selected Essays of William Hazlitt
Introduced by Duncan Wu